THE HEALTHCARE CRISIS:

The Urgent Need for Physician Leadership

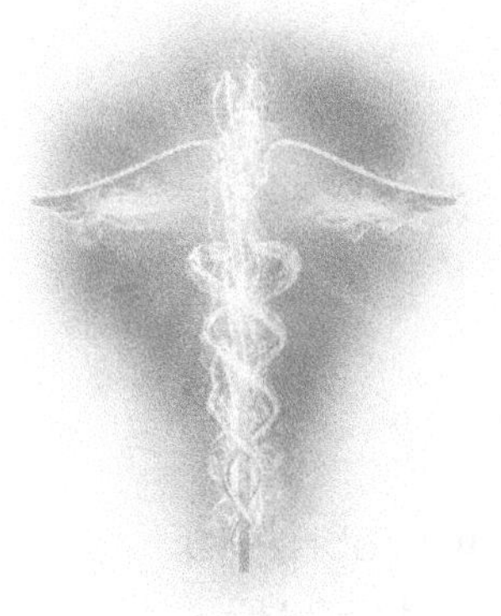

Fredric Tobis, MD

Published in 2012.
Center for Physician Leadership Training
Mercer Island, WA
cfplt.com

ISBN-10: 1477640479
EAN-13: 9781477640470

Editorial services provided by:
Rebecca Buffum Taylor, Prose/Arts
prose.arts@gmail.com

For Carla Joy,
The beacon in my life.

Contents

Introduction
An insider's point of view

A number of complex issues – social, moral, fiscal, legal – have become tightly entangled in the American healthcare crisis, but however deeply rooted and chaotic, all lead back to the central problem: skyrocketing costs. There is no other more urgent problem in healthcare today. To succeed in the long run, workable healthcare reform must focus on resolving our country's out-of-control, unsustainable costs. Health care is hemorrhaging massively and bleeding into other national issues, from the federal budget deficit to losing competitive viability in the global marketplace.

The time has passed to hope that minor fixes imposed from outside of the healthcare system will work. Instead, it's time to focus on how to resolve national healthcare spending with a major revamping from within.

For the past 25 years, I have been intricately involved in efforts to improve the quality and efficiency of our healthcare system. My efforts began with a successful, Seattle-based group cardiology practice and expanded in the past 10 years as an independent healthcare and physician leadership consultant. During this time, I've worked with a wide range of providers and insurers throughout the country, sharing the frustrations they have all repeatedly expressed about the inequality, inefficiency, and instability of our current healthcare system, along with the multiple failures of an increasingly burdensome regulatory environment to address those issues.

I've also had the opportunity to travel regularly to our nation's capital and talk with members of Congress from Washington State. I've come to understand a great deal more about how the political process works, from where Congress obtains its massive amount of information to make decisions to the formidable time constraints under which those decisions are made. Sitting in Congressional offices, coming to know members of Congress and their staffs over time, has given me an invaluable inside perspective about how things really work in D.C.

The Congress members I've met see themselves as civil servants trying to make a difference. Their lives are incredibly stressful; they're on the plane constantly commuting between their home districts and Capitol Hill, running political campaigns while they're processing the enormous amounts of data required to understand the nuances of bills coming up for vote, from health care to the environment, the military, the mortgage industry, and the budget deficit.

Given the complexity of health care, the limited availability of truly objective data, and the time demands on our members of Congress, it's no surprise that the healthcare crisis remains unsolved. What puzzles me is that while Congress has been actively trying to solve the healthcare crisis, we physicians have remained largely on the sidelines, remarkably passive. Congress proposes; we react. In essence, we've been asking the cart to lead the horse, and it's unfair to Congress and to our country's healthcare consumers. As physicians, I believe that it's part of our responsibility to our profession to lead the development of value-driven solutions to our healthcare crisis that Congress and an informed public can then respond to, secure in the knowledge that those solutions have a good chance of actually working clinically, on the ground.

In 2008, I was asked by Congressman Dave Reichert to chair Washington State's Eighth Congressional District Health Care Advisory

Committee. Since then, at our quarterly meetings, I've facilitated discussions among a diverse group of local healthcare leaders representing major medical centers, physician groups, biotech companies, private insurers, and the large state-funded and federally funded programs. We are, in essence, a combination of a focus group and town hall meeting for health care.

The last four quarterly meetings have, not surprisingly, focused on the potential impact on our medical community of implementing the Affordable Care Act of 2010. In our meetings, after each member reported on the implications of the new healthcare legislation for their specific institution or customers, we challenged ourselves to look beyond our parochial issues with the Affordable Care Act and focus rather on its effect on the more far-reaching issues facing our healthcare system. It soon became clear to me that the knowledge base and creativity of the providers and payers in the room, and in similar rooms throughout the nation, could yield a more powerful, long-term impact by proactively forming healthcare policy rather than reacting to the inadequacies of current, politically driven policies.

With this book, by taking a deeper look behind the scenes into the world of physicians and the hospitals in which they practice today, I hope to reveal the hard truths hidden behind the media sound bites that distort the current healthcare debate. I hope to paint a more accurate picture of the healthcare landscape that provides enough background and context to understand the key issues in the reform debate – as well as to reframe the debate in a more viable way that leads to a lasting solution. Only by facing today's on-the-ground realities and asking the tough questions can we resolve the healthcare crisis in a way that preserves the best of what American medicine has to offer and provides the most beneficial long-term outcome for all.

It's my hope that consumers, as well as fellow physicians, hospital leadership, and politicians, will find this insider's voice a useful guide to the ongoing dialog on healthcare reform, one that's balanced, fair-minded, and seeks a path toward win-win solutions. Regardless of who serves in Congress or the Oval Office in the foreseeable future, consumers will be called upon repeatedly to vote on healthcare issues in local political elections, in national elections – and with their pocketbooks. By better understanding the realities behind the sound bites on those issues, consumers can make a difference in the future of American health care. New paradigms and policies driven by thoughtful healthcare providers can lead our country toward a system that's both high quality and affordable – health care that demonstrates value. The creation of this value proposition will require the support of well-informed consumers as well as the ongoing creativity, responsibility, and perseverance of effective physician leaders.

Chapter 1
The Urgent Crisis: Spiraling Costs

Healthcare spending and GDP

Total spending for U.S. health care is a constantly moving target. One recent estimate from the Centers for Medicare and Medicaid Services (CMS) predicts that total healthcare spending will double from $2.6 trillion in 2010 to $4.6 trillion in 2020 – and to reach 20% of our gross domestic product, or GDP, by 2020. To put that into an historical context, healthcare spending was only 4.7% of GDP in 1960.

Using this measure – percentage of gross domestic product – is the most objective way to understand healthcare spending. The higher the percentage of GDP spent on any one line item in a country's budget, the less economically viable that country is in the global marketplace. Since we're currently spending 17.6% of our GDP on health care and our global competitors are averaging 9%, American businesses falter at an economic disadvantage in the global market; they're spending much more than their competitors on a fixed cost.

Percentage of GDP is also a useful gauge showing that spending an inordinate amount of money on health care leaves less funding for education, infrastructure, social services, and other essential expenses.

GDP as a global benchmark, then, allows countries to compare costs across a global community within a consistent framework. In addition, by definition, as a society grows, costs grow; and GDP gives everyone a relative basis for comparison.

In the last half of this century, healthcare spending has skyrocketed, from 4% of gross domestic product in 1950, to 12% in 1990, to nearly 18% now. Without correcting for growth, economists see skewed trends over time, so they've developed sophisticated algorithms for evaluating those trends. But from an overall global perspective, when you look at various societies and what they're spending on health care as a percentage of their GDP, it tells you a lot about their priorities compared to other countries. The urgency now is that Americans may not recognize that we're spending too much money on health care until we approach spending 25%, 30%, or 40% of our GDP on that one line item in our national budget.

There's a tipping point in healthcare spending where costs will be shifted so much onto patients and businesses that they'll simply push for a single-party-payer system to correct the crisis. Many business leaders are already there; they're fatigued from trying so many different ways to control their healthcare costs that have been uniformly unsuccessful. In addition, the amount of money consumers spend every year out-of-pocket for medical expenses grows every year. As a consumer, you might tolerate spending 10% of your income on health care, but would you tolerate spending 50%? If our country doesn't do something in the near future, that could easily happen; by then the crisis will be even more urgent to fix, and the only quick fix is a single-party payer. That's the fastest, easiest way to control healthcare spending; even people who argue against a single-party payer agree with that point. The one thing that Canada, England, and others with a single-party payer can do: they can control their healthcare costs. Those countries say they'll spend 10% or other percentage of their GDP on health care, and when that money runs out, they essentially stop spending.

Another reason to evaluate national healthcare costs as a percentage of GDP is that we're still hiding healthcare costs behind deficit spending, so instead of having a "100% mindset," we just keep on spending and borrowing from other parts of the federal budget. The federal government is tapping into the Medicare trust fund to pay for current healthcare overutilization, so we're not just overspending money this year, we're deficit spending with money that was put away to keep the country solvent. It's the difference between paying off bills at the end of the month and using a credit card; as a country we've been going into major debt to support the current system. Medicare is not balancing its budget; it's losing money and drawing off the Medicare trust fund with the assumption that the trust fund will grow again in the future.

GDP is an indicator of how expensive health care is in this country. It shows how we're spending our money and what the trends are. It's ironic that people grow angry about defense spending, when we're spending less than 4% of our GDP on defense. By comparison, we're spending an incredible amount of money on health care – but are we getting value? Somewhere there's a more rational balance to achieve a healthy, viable society as well as be competitive in the global market.

Medicare: the elephant in the room

The Centers for Medicare & Medicaid (CMS) has predicted that by 2020, healthcare spending per capita will jump to over $13,000, up from over $8,000 in 2010. CMS also projects that Medicare spending alone will rise nearly 7% per year from 2009 to 2019, and Medicaid spending will rise nearly 8% per year during that same period.

Medicare began in 1965 with a fairly modest budget, but its budget has been growing exponentially and is about to explode. All U.S. citizens and lawfully admitted immigrants are eligible for Medicare when they reach age 65. When Medicare started, the average life expectancy in the United States was just over 70 years; in 2009 it was over 78. Figures from the 1960 census showed that back then, only about 17 million Americans, or 9% of the total population, were over 65 and therefore Medicare eligible. In the 2010 census, 40 million Americans, or 13%, were over 65. Further, the census projections for growth indicate that in 2050, 89 million seniors, or 20% of the U.S. population, will be Medicare-eligible under current criteria.

According to the nonpartisan Congressional Budget Office (CBO), total spending for Medicare and Medicaid increased from 1.7% of GDP in fiscal year 1975 to 5.7% in fiscal year 2008. Federal spending alone (excluding state spending) for the two programs increased from 1.2% to 4.1% of GDP. The same CBO report predicts that, without significant policy changes, total Medicare spending alone is projected to increase to 8% of GDP by 2035 and to 15% by 2080.

Out-of-control spending – not access, not universal coverage, not privacy, portability, electronic medical records, or any of the other single, hotly debated, media sound bites in health care – is the issue. Creating real value in health care is the solution, and physicians, not politicians, should be charged with solving the problem. This is the mission behind my work with physician leadership: Doctors remain the vital untapped resource in how to use healthcare dollars most effectively for the greatest value. The current system – most notably Medicare – simply can't continue to add extra expenses and minor fixes that hide the real issues driving the escalating costs of health care.

Almost by definition, then, reforming health care means changing Medicare. Medicare is the single biggest player in the third-party-payer system (where a third party pays for medical care rendered to consumers). Medicare is also the shield behind which all other insurance companies hide. If Medicare tries something and it seems to work, the other players follow suit, rather than testing new ideas in the marketplace themselves where they stand to lose customers and revenue. Most professionals in medicine would agree: As goes Medicare, so goes health care.

Medicare is also the most strategic player because we can't solve health care – and can't balance the budget or pull the country out of the quicksand we're in with deficit spending – without addressing

Medicare. Most healthcare economists would agree that everything else pales in comparison when it comes to health care. Medicare is the largest, growing, unfunded entitlement program our country has, constantly borrowing money from its trust fund to keep itself afloat for years. Medicare will run out of funds in the near or very-near future, depending on which economist does the analysis. Some economists who define bankruptcy as "borrowing from the public trust fund" say that Medicare is "bankrupt" now; others say it will be bankrupt by 2024.

In all probability, American lifespans will continue to lengthen in the future. Medicare began at a time when the number of elderly was a relatively small portion of the population. Now that the first baby boomers have entered the Medicare system, we'll continue to have a huge number of retirees who are not paying taxes but are supported by tax-payer revenue – in essence, riding on the back of a much smaller number of workers who are putting money into the system. Given the current economy, the upcoming generation may earn incomes lower than the Medicare beneficiaries enjoy through their retiree benefits, stocks, and other income.

It's worth asking whether we as a society want to continue to pay ex-vice presidents and ex-CEOs their Medicare benefits. They're eligible to receive benefits, but should they be? The question is part of the process of redefining health care in this new era, and doing the hard work of rethinking and possibly redesigning certain entitlements. Theoretically, an ex-CEO today could be in the hospital for bypass surgery being paid for by the guy who mows his lawn.

The cost to business: America's global disadvantage

Our current healthcare system clearly puts American businesses at a disadvantage in the global market. As an example: The aircraft manufacturer Boeing pays a significant percentage of its overhead for health insurance for its employees, while its global competitor, Airbus, pays no direct health insurance costs since France has socialized medicine. Boeing is at a clear disadvantage, costing our country jobs. We can't compete in the global market when we're the only country in the first world sustaining healthcare costs at the rate that we're sustaining them.

The nonpartisan Kaiser Health News reported that employers saw a surge of 9% in the cost of providing health coverage for their workers in 2011, triple the rise in their costs over 2010. The annual, employer-sponsored health plan premiums in 2011 alone cost employers an average of $15,073 for family plans and $5,429 for individual plans. General Motors provides healthcare benefits to 1.1 million employees and retirees, spending $5 billion a year on healthcare costs; it adds an average of $2,000 to the sticker price of every new car to pay for this, putting the company at a significant disadvantage when competing with European or Asian car manufacturers whose workers are covered by national healthcare systems.

When you look at the current debate on the federal budget, it's clear that it doesn't matter what you do with taxation; if you don't fix the deficit, it's irrelevant – and the ultimate problem with the deficit is Medicare. No one likes to talk about it, but it's not sustainable, and for a variety of reasons. We've gotten into this mess because we've never been able to ask: What is a reasonable healthcare package that we as society should pay for, what should individuals be responsible for, and how do we balance those? Who ought to receive benefits and who ought to pay for their own? How do we define value in health care? What new technologies add value, and not just cost?

Instead of asking the tough questions, we've essentially said that everyone insured is eligible for everything. Imagine expanding your home budget to include your extended family and their friends and neighbors, and allowing them all to purchase everything they wanted. No matter how hard you worked, you'd be out in the street in no time. At some point our healthcare policies need to resolve the competing values of universal coverage and no "caps" on spending with the financial realities of medicine today.

Overutilization drives spiraling costs

The pressing issue with health care today is overall cost, and the problem with cost is not physicians' salaries, nurses' salaries, or lab techs' salaries; it's overutilization.

Why in the United States do we spend more than twice as much per capita on health care than any other nation in the 30-country Organisation for Economic Co-operation and Development (OECD), a group of the most economically advanced democracies in the world? Why do we perform almost twice the average number of coronary revascularizations (open heart surgeries and angioplasties) than anywhere else in the world? We've created a system that rewards the use of expensive, high-tech procedures, tests, and technologies – and penalizes physicians financially for spending time with patients. These hidden financial incentives in medicine drive utilization – and overutilization.

According to a study published in 2007 by the nonpartisan Congressional Research Service, the number of MRI units per one million people among the most economically advanced countries in the world averaged 8.8 in 2004, compared to 26.6 in the United States in that same year. Canadian physicians, for instance, order far fewer surgeries, high-tech procedures, and tests than physicians in our country. Granted, they have a different population, with less violent crime, fewer teenage single mothers, and different societal expectations of health care, but that doesn't fully explain the variation. It's not that Canada avoids doing open-heart surgeries or echocardiograms. But when a Canadian province receives its budget for the year, its leaders have to be careful how they manage that money to allocate for all of their needs, from education and transportation to health care, because they know there's a fixed cap on their spending.

The biggest cost – utilization – is hidden

When I'm sitting in a room with CEOs, CFOs, and COOs of corporate America, I ask them, "When you look at your quarterly financials, how many of you have a spreadsheet that doesn't reflect the biggest overall cost to your organization?" They looked stunned and incredulous. They can't imagine running a successful business that way – exactly the way health care is run.

The reality is that in a typical board-of-directors' meeting in a hospital, when they look at their spreadsheets, they don't have data for their biggest cost: healthcare utilization. The real drivers behind overall costs are the utilization patterns, which are primarily driven by physicians. The hospital spreadsheet doesn't account for that reality. Instead, the hospital board is looking at nursing salaries, bills for electricity, salaries for administrative and janitorial staff, depreciation tables, interest burdens, and other financial factors. But they're not seeing that Dr. Lean admits a patient to the hospital and discharges him in one day, while Dr. Chubb admits the same type of patient and keeps him there for a week.

Hospital leaders began to track utilization data such as length-of-stay in the hospital and other measures of efficiency in the 1980s, with the introduction of the prospective payment system based on diagnosis-related groupings, or DRGs. Prospective payments are a form of prepayment to a hospital that have a cap: Caring for this patient will earn the hospital a set fee and no more. When you're a hospital receiving prospective payment for your patients, it only makes sense to stay keenly attentive to how all of the physicians on your staff use your hospital resources. You're likely to have some doctors who work efficiently in how they utilize the hospital's resources – they basically provide good "value" – and other doctors who may achieve reasonable medical outcomes but at ten times the cost to the hospital. The financial spreadsheets aren't showing this.

Hospital boards of directors don't have that data, so they're often unaware of the problem. Granted, actionable data in this arena is difficult to collect. Several doctors are often involved with the care of hospitalized patients, making it difficult to attribute costs accurately to each of them. The electronic medical records systems currently in use don't have the capability of accurate accounting for costs in terms of the number of physician visits per patient, length of time per visit, time spent with families, and other cost factors.

Even if accurate data were available, it would be hard to work with it constructively because of the longstanding history of hospitals' relationships with their doctors. To strip a physician of admitting privileges because of utilization patterns would be extremely difficult, because doctors will always argue that they alone have the right to determine quality of care. In fact, they have legal protection regarding that determination. Even if a hospital took the legal risk to try to strip a doctor of privileges, its risk of negative publicity would be substantial. The media would have a field day with negative sound bites: "Local hospital fires physician for spending too much money taking care of patients." The negative spin and the legal battles make it almost impossible for a hospital to ask a physician with unsound utilization practices to leave and practice somewhere else.

So how do most hospitals try to control their costs? They cut the expenses they can measure and control. They start slashing nursing budgets, so patients in a hospital ring their bells at night for a nurse and experience an increasingly slow response or, too often, no response at all.

Similarly, the skyrocketing costs of Medicare don't stem from physician reimbursement; that's akin to looking at nurses' salaries on a hospital's operating spreadsheet and thinking that's the line item to focus on. The problem is not what we're paying nurses or doctors to see patients, but what doctors cost the system through Medicare-incentivized utilization of high-tech testing, diagnostic imaging, expensive surgeries and procedures, hospital resources, and other healthcare costs.

The Medicare Payment Advisory Committee agrees that overutilization of resources, driven primarily by specialists under the economic incentives of the current reimbursement scheme, forces future Medicare cuts that hurt primary care providers disproportionately. A system called the Resource-Based Relative Value Scale weighs various physician services, from surgery to time spent with patients in office visits; not surprisingly, high-tech, complex, specialty procedures and diagnostic testing win out. They're "valued" higher on the resource scale – and therefore they reimburse more than a primary care doctor's consult with a patient.

Every time my elderly aunt goes to see her Medicare doctor, for instance, he orders a chest x-ray, a blood test, or an EKG – with a frequency not indicated for her condition. She recently told me she was anemic. No wonder she's anemic; every time she sees her doctor, he's drawing more blood. The current system of reimbursement incentivizes even simple, repeated testing as a way to boost flagging incomes.

Medicaid and Medicare reimbursement realities

Consumers may think about Medicaid and Medicare as if they're similar, but they've always been vastly different, especially from the physicians' perspective. From the beginning, Medicaid has never adequately reimbursed doctors or hospitals. Medicaid, which primarily covers the poor, is still considered a form of charity by many people. Medicare, on the other hand, is still considered an earned entitlement.

Because Medicaid has never adequately reimbursed physicians, the only physicians who were actually profitable taking Medicaid patients were the ones running "Medicaid factories," where they were seeing a patient every few minutes or ordering frequent lab testing. Otherwise, what Medicaid pays doesn't cover most physicians' overhead and expenses to see those patients, so the doctors lose money. Very few doctors, in all honesty, want to take on Medicaid patients; most do it out of moral obligation or for personal reasons, not because they can make a living doing it.

Another major difference between the two public insurance programs arises from political clout. Medicaid covers poor people and their dependents as well as disabled people, populations that tend to have little political influence; people living near poverty level tend not to vote or access their local politicians. Medicare, on the other hand, covers those with an increasingly large demographic footprint, the financial resources to have their own powerful lobby (AARP), and the passionate political interest that consistently turns out votes in numbers disproportionately large to their already large demographics. Woe to the politician who crosses swords with American seniors.

Robbing Peter to pay Paul: cutting reimbursement to doctors

To add insult to injury for physicians, already low reimbursements for Medicaid and Medicare patients are in constant jeopardy of further cuts each year. Part of the federal Balanced Budget Act of 1997 added a formula for controlling Medicare's payments to physicians, called the sustainable growth rate (SGR) formula, which critics contend not only has inherent issues in itself but also wasn't calculated into the costs of the healthcare reform legislation of 2010. The SGR tied doctors' fees to growth in GDP and a balanced federal budget, so that Medicare Part B spending for physicians' services wouldn't outstrip a set percentage of increase in GDP.

Since its inception, the SGR authorized cuts in physician reimbursement whenever the Medicare budget wasn't adequately supported by federal revenue. According to the Center on Budget and Policy Priorities, by 2002 the SGR formula had cut physician payments by nearly 5%. Fearing that further reductions in physician reimbursement would jeopardize Medicare beneficiaries' access to care, Congress has effectively stepped in since 2003 and prevented the full SGR cuts from happening. But the SGR formula, still on the books, advises a deeper cut into physician reimbursement each year, and by 2010 proposed that physician payment rates be cut by a whopping 21.2%. The costs associated with resolving the SGR issue and reinstating appropriate physician pay for services already deeply cut – costs that are separate from any healthcare reform laws already passed or enacted in the future – still needs to be addressed.

Congressional concerns over Medicare patients' access to care are far from unfounded. When Medicare patients could no longer afford medications that were becoming ridiculously expensive, the government added Plan D, which extended prescription benefits for Medicare patients. With Plan D, Medicare patients have co-pays, but they're small; the federal budget essentially pays the bulk of the cost for their medications.

How did government pay for the drug benefit? They robbed Peter (physicians) to pay Paul (the pharmaceutical industry). While the public may assume that the government was playing a shell game and borrowing against some other line item in the federal budget, in fact they cut reimbursement to physicians through the sustainable growth rate formula (SGR) to pay for the drug benefit. Certain specialties – primary care physicians in particular – were hit hard. My elderly aunt, for instance, now has all of her medications paid for, but she struggles to find a physician who'll take her on as a Medicare patient. More doctors, especially those in primary care, are opting out of the Medicare system entirely because the reimbursements are so low. The independent panel that advises Congress on Medicare, the Medicare Payment Advisory Committee, reported in 2008 that nearly one-third of patients entitled to Medicare had difficulty finding a doctor willing to treat them.

Currently, the argument continues about "sustainable growth" in Medicare Part B for physicians' services. Since 1997, under the SGR limits, physicians' fees were scheduled for cuts several times – and several times Congress, under pressure from physician lobbies, intervened to block SGR reductions; but the latest federal budget called for 29% mandated cuts in physician services. Imagine the push-back if other American professionals were asked to cut their salaries by nearly one-third.

Some groups of fiscal conservatives want to limit the growth of Medicare spending by maintaining the SGR limits. They simply want to cap Medicare spending, but that's not addressing the real problems: fee-for-service reimbursement and overutilization. The physician lobbyists tell everyone on Capitol Hill to vote to repeal the SGR limits, which would allow doctors to make more money, arguing that the SGR is choking off health care – and, under today's dysfunctional reimbursement system, they're right. Those physicians who are poorly reimbursed by today's fee structures are retiring early; they can't make ends meet. On the other hand, without a sustainable growth rate clause in Medicare under the current fee-for-service system, it guarantees that healthcare spending will continue to explode, and it's already at an unsustainable level.

The amount of money needed to keep Medicare up and running is enormous, beautifully illustrated in a cartoon comparing the funding needed to service Medicare with the amount needed to service the national deficit. The caption asks, "Are you worried about the national deficit? Don't worry about it." The cartoon shows two spheres, side by side: The national deficit is the size of a baseball, while Medicare is the size of the Earth.

Understanding DRGs versus fee-for-service

When healthcare costs continued to rise rapidly through the 1960s and 1970s after the advent of medical insurance, Medicare began to grow nervous. By the 1980s, Medicare started taking a serious look at their costs. The Jeremiahs – the "weeping prophets" – started saying, "Medicare tomorrow will not be your father's or grandfather's Medicare." They saw that Medicare was dealing with a radical new set of dynamics driven by increased life expectancy, which had risen significantly after the release of new medical technology. Given the ability to keep people alive longer – sometimes long after they want to live – and the aging baby boomer demographic, they realized that the population covered by Medicare was about to explode in numbers. The country's healthcare system, they feared, would collapse under its weight.

So Medicare did something smart in 1982: It looked at hospital fees and came up with the idea of DRGs, or diagnosis-related groups, as a way to control its own costs. Why focus on hospital fees? In a typical bill for hospitalization, more than two-thirds of what's charged to patients constitutes hospital fees, with the rest divided into physician fees, pharmacy fees, medical equipment such as wheelchairs, and other hospitalization-related fees. Medicare used a common-sense approach to control its spending, much like looking at any other spreadsheet: When you try to cut costs, you start with your biggest expenditures.

Because they were paying their biggest bills to hospitals for hospitalization, Medicare came up with the idea of starting to pay prospectively for care, instead of paying the "usual and customary" rates. The new DRG system was a prospective payment system, where Medicare and hospitals agreed on a set fee for providing care to each of the hundreds of DRG categories of patients before any care was actually given. In contrast, traditional fee-for-service is a retrospective payment system, where doctors and hospitals send bills to insurers and receive payment after care has been given and its costs incurred to the patient and the system overall. Diagnosis-related groups were originally developed for the Health Care Financing Administration as a way not only to group similar patients by their diagnoses and treatment needs but also to relate a hospital's "case mix" of patients to its costs and resource needs. Close to 600 DRG codes now exist, and each can represent an expected profit margin or loss to a hospital.

More and more effort today is being made to prepay, or bundle, services rather than pay hospitals with the old fee-for-service system, which essentially paid piecemeal for every lab test, procedure, patient contact, and hospital resource or service used. Many policy experts believe that prepaying hospitals via bundled services will eventually trickle down to the physician community, but so far doctors have been able to avoid it, primarily through strong lobbying efforts by their specialty groups in D.C. Physicians, for the most part, are still in the fee-for-service mode.

The fee-for-service payment system remains as a vestige of the preinsurance era, when patients paid providers directly for services rendered. This economic model has validity when a consumer pays a vendor for a service. In the past, both patients and physicians had economic incentives to keep fees reasonable, and physicians would often negotiate their fees, set on a sliding scale depending on a patient's ability to pay, or even barter with patients for services. The validity of the fee-for-service model disappears when the patient receives a service from a physician that is paid for primarily by a third party, such as an insurer, where there's little economic incentive to reach and maintain reasonable fees.

Initially, health insurance, including Medicare, continued the traditional fee-for-service method of payment to both hospitals and physicians. With the institution of DRGs, though, Medicare eliminated fee-for-service payments to hospitals in Medicare Part A but continued to pay physicians in Medicare Part B in the fee-for-service mode. Eventually, Medicare changed the fee structure for physicians from a "usual and customary fee" set by the physician to a preset fee determined by the detailed formula known as the Resource-Based Relative Value Scale. But today, all doctors, even those working in HMOs and other employment models, bill Medicare Part B for their physicians' services on a fee-for-service basis.

Medicare now pays hospitals via predetermined, bundled payments for all costs incurred during a hospital admission for a given diagnosis-related group. This Medicare-initiated, bundled payment system has been copied by Medicaid and almost all private insurers, although it's not used for uninsured, self-pay patients. Hospitals in a given region receive the same reimbursement for the same DRG code, with the exception of university hospitals, which may be reimbursed at a slightly higher rate as teaching hospitals with a large volume of low-income patients.

Differences exist among geographic regions – what a Seattle hospital receives versus a San Francisco or New York hospital – and that, too, is complicated, and based on history and tradition. When DRGs came into play, Medicare looked at what they had spent in the past several years on each primary diagnosis, such as congestive heart failure or kidney disease, and they noticed regional variations. Their analysis was that the variation reflected regional differences in labor costs. They then picked an amount they thought was a reasonable prepayment based on trends and on an assumption that the Northeast has higher labor costs and should receive a higher DRG payment.

The reality is that factors other than labor costs contributed to regional variations, including an incredible amount of inefficiency and differences in style in how physicians practice. There's an ongoing, heated debate now about whether to do away with regional differences. In an effort to save money, one could argue that if the West Coast traditionally has the lowest utilization rate and the most efficient way of taking care of patients with certain DRGs, that that should be the standard protocol, and everyone else needs to figure out how to follow it. But in Congress and especially in the House, where there are many more representatives from Pennsylvania than from Washington State, it would be a political battle to adopt that idea.

DRG payments in a given region are basically consistent – as are fee-for-service diagnostic and procedural reimbursement rates. An insurer such as Premera negotiates with physicians and sets their rates, which depend on how big their group practice is and how much clout those docs have. Physicians at a large, respected, city hospital might be able to negotiate a higher reimbursement with Premera than a doctor in solo practice. But regardless of the payer, physicians are still billing on a fee-for-service basis – that's the issue. Because doctors are billing fee-for-service at a predetermined discount rate, the more services they provide, the higher their reimbursement. If a patient spends unnecessary time in the hospital or receives unnecessary testing by a physician in the hospital, the doctor does better financially – while the hospital and the overall system suffer.

When Medicare and hospitals began using DRGs, before the hospitals started "playing the payer mix," the first thing they did was to analyze more closely the waste within the hospital system. The idea of "utilization review" didn't start until prospective payments started with DRGs, forcing hospital leaders to realize they'd better get a handle on how to manage their costs quickly. True, hospitals do push physicians to discharge patients and send them home quicker because of DRGs, but there's still unnecessary variation in the care and associated costs of care among physicians, which is currently not included in the bundled payment. At this point, American doctors have no economic incentive to be efficient within the hospital; they're essentially going to get paid every time they touch a patient. The well-accepted principle that unexplained and unnecessary "variation in production" leads to increased cost and decreased quality has been embraced by other industries – airlines, car manufacturers, and high-tech industries – but not by health care.

Physicians and the culture of autonomy

The relationship between physicians and hospitals has always been incredibly complex. From 1751, with the founding of Pennsylvania Hospital by Ben Franklin and Thomas Bond, MD, physicians were independent contractors who applied for privileges at a given hospital and were essentially guaranteed privileges to practice there. Later, with the advent of standardized, scientific medical education in the United States after the American Medical Association spearheaded the publication of the Flexner Report in 1910, the criteria for hospitals to grant privileges to physicians were based on credentialing: A doctor had to have graduated from an accredited medical school and completed supervised postgraduate training. From the hospital's standpoint, the more credentialed physicians it had practicing on staff, the higher the patient volume and revenue it could earn as a hospital.

So in the classic tradition of medicine, physicians don't have a boss; as physicians, we see the boss every day in the mirror when we get dressed. We're selected, educated, and indoctrinated to be autonomous decision-makers. Physicians live in this deeply engrained mindset of autonomy, whether they become independent members of a medical staff, members of group practices, members of a foundation-style hospital, or a hospital employee. This culture of autonomy has never been a great fit for hospitals, which depend on staff to function in a collaborative mode, but while the hospitals' algorithm for success was to fill their beds, the autonomous culture was tolerated. Because hospitals have always been dependent on doctors for their referrals and therefore their revenue, hospital leadership couldn't tell physicians, "That test you ordered isn't really necessary; you need to do your patient rounds more than once a day because we need to get patients out of the hospital as soon as possible; and by the way, your colleagues here typically spend half of the hospital resources that you spend, so straighten up and fly right."

Hospitals have always had trouble controlling physician behavior because of the long history of the complicated financial relationship between the two groups. In many ways they depend on each other financially and support each other, but in other ways they're competing with each other for their own piece of the healthcare pie. There are legal and regulatory ties as well. Physicians censored by hospitals can use the restraint-of-trade argument, and physicians under review can claim that their censorship was motivated by other physicians' competition and economic greed. When a physician is clearly incompetent, it's a logistical nightmare for a hospital to try to remove that physician from its staff; and when a physician provides well-below-par quality of care, it's still nearly impossible.

The bottom line: You can't control hospital costs without controlling physician autonomy. If physicians have no financial accountability for how they do things, it's impossible to control hospital costs.

The love/hate relationship with hospitals and physicians

The relationship between hospitals and physicians is the ultimate love/hate relationship, complicated further by continually changing regulations. The way hospitals made a profit prior to the DRG system was by keeping all their beds filled, so they got the "biggest bang out of their buck" from the staff since they were charging whatever their costs were plus a percentage for profit. The higher the volume of patients, the better.

Hospitals went out of their way to put as many doctors on staff as possible and to woo those doctors with high patient loads – the source of patients to fill beds – with a variety of special benefits. Hospitals looked at the physicians as their "customers," since physicians are who brought patients into the hospital. They wooed busy doctors onto the hospital staff with plush doctors' lounges, complimentary food and beverages, free designated parking, blocked time for their procedure scheduling, and an overhead-free environment in which to work. In some ways, both hospitals and doctors are still stuck in that mode.

The current legal environment binds hospitals to doctors even further. Today, once a physician has privileges at a hospital, it's extremely difficult for the hospital to rescind them. Once a physician is on staff at a hospital, unless that person engages in obviously egregious behavior, it's unlikely that the hospital will be able to remove that physician from the staff; and even if the hospital is successful, it's likely to cost a fortune in legal fees. Doctors wanting to maintain their medical staff privileges at a hospital are further protected by federal and state mandates, so hospitals dealing with below-par physicians or those trying to rank physicians' economic performance face huge challenges due to poor data on physician utilization as well as legal requirements that prevent interference with physician judgment. This dilemma alone illuminates how unique the healthcare environment is, compared to other businesses where employers have a high degree of control and authority over the people who work for them and an accurate way of measuring and controlling their business costs.

Hospital discharge summaries represent a classic operational conflict between hospitals and physicians. Physicians can bill for their services as soon as the patient leaves the hospital. Hospitals can't bill Medicare for patient care until a physician dictates a discharge summary and that discharge summary has been verified and signed by that doctor to ensure that it's correct and there's no "missed diagnosis" or "mis-diagnosis." If you miss a diagnosis, you miss a reimbursement, so the hospital loses money. If you miscode a diagnosis, both the hospital and the treating physician can be legally punished because it's considered "Medicare fraud and abuse." The unfunny joke here is that many "Medicare fraud and abuse" cases are honest provider mistakes with complicated codes and criteria that keep changing all the time, but politicians create sound bites around "Medicare fraud and abuse" to imply that they're going to save the country billions of dollars by going after the "fraud and abuse" providers.

The relationship between hospitals and their medical staffs is starting to change, but it's changing slowly. Hospitals are now moving to a new model where a foundation owns the hospital and its group physician practices, or to direct ownership/employment models in which a hospital employs its physicians, where permitted by state law. Unfortunately, even in these more progressive models, efforts to move into truly integrated, collaborative models are hindered by hidden financial incentives, burdensome regulations, and the longstanding physician mindset of autonomy.

The new hospital profit model

DRGs and other forms of global payments for services have changed the hospital's financial algorithm for success. The algorithm has shifted from simply filling beds to three critical strategies, all of which present a challenge to the culture of physician autonomy.

- **Optimize the payer mix.** Hospitals welcome patients with private insurance, get by with patients on Medicare, and try to limit Medicaid and the uninsured due to high default rates on their billings.
- **Maximize profitable DRG admissions.** Cardiovascular surgery, cardiology, oncology, orthopedics, and neurosurgery all represent potential profit to the hospital due to their high utilization of relatively well-reimbursed technology and procedures.
- **Minimize resource utilization.** Hospitals try to control their use of in-house resources and costs for DRGs that typically cost them money, such as elderly patients with pneumonia.

The algorithm for hospitals' financial success has therefore shifted from welcoming all physicians to apply for staff privileges to recruiting cardiac surgeons, cardiologists, oncologists, neurosurgeons, and orthopedic surgeons, hoping to attract their profitable DRG admissions. Their patients typically undergo well-reimbursed procedures and short length of stays in the hospital. Conversely, hospital leadership is less enamoured of attracting doctors who take care of patients whose DRG admissions have a high likelihood of a negative cash flow, such as elderly patients with pneumonia, renal failure, and other chronic diseases, who often need lengthy hospitalizations and offer no procedural profits.

A perfect "recruitment wave" forms when a profitable procedure meets an efficient physician. Cardiac stenting is a good example of such a perfect wave. Stenting is pretty well reimbursed by all payers and, when performed by efficient cardiologists, quite profitable. Even after *The New England Journal of Medicine* published a landmark 2007 study casting doubt on the viability and benefits of stenting, hospitals continue to recruit cardiologists, and Medicare continues to spend huge sums reimbursing the procedure. It's especially profitable for the hospital when its cardiologists can agree to use the cheapest stents, limit the number of stents used, and discharge patients rapidly.

An example of this recruitment wave was exposed during an investigation by the Senate Finance Committee, which oversees Medicare. The Committee investigated a Baltimore-area cardiologist, heavily recruited by the hospital in which he worked, who had performed 30 stent procedures in one day, and concluded that he "may have implanted 585 stents which were medically unnecessary" between 2007 and 2009. As *The New York Times* reported on the case on December 5, 2010: "Medicare paid $3.8 million of the $6.6 million charged for those procedures," and, even more sobering, spent $3.5 *billion* on stent procedures in 2009 alone.

Perverse incentives: winners and losers in medicine

The current fee-for-service reimbursement paradigm has created an unprecedented disparity in income among healthcare providers and has pitted primary care doctors against specialists, specialists against one another, hospitals against physicians, and physicians and hospitals against insurers. The income disparity and outright competition translates into disparate goals and disparate power and influence in achieving those goals. This is balkanized medicine.

Winners and losers appear in the system. Some specialties – and therefore some patients – win big; others lose big. Cardiac patients, for instance, are treated well by the system. They often see specialists in upscale institutions, with budgets for fancy carpets, expensive artwork, and dedicated nurses who call them at home and provide extra, hands-on care. Orthopedic suites tend to be upscale, too, thanks to all the arthroscopies and joint replacement surgeries that orthopedic surgeons now perform. The problem, from a national policy perspective and overall cost standpoint, is that these expenditures may not make the most sense in terms of using national healthcare dollars to add the most value.

The physician community is still divided about the fee-for-service model that has led to balkanized medicine. Primary care doctors, who have been the most severely squeezed financially since the measures moving toward a federal balanced budget amendment and sustained growth rate (SGR) formulas were adopted, generally look forward to the end of fee-for-service. Their views are shared by some specialists, such as general surgeons, who have also been squeezed, although many specialists who are still doing well financially with fee-for-service are reluctant to see the system change. A huge gap remains in annual earnings between primary care doctors and specialists. In 2008, according to the federal Bureau of Labor Statistics, primary care doctors earned a median annual income of about $186,000, while specialists earned nearly $340,000.

The supposed cure for the problem – cutting back physician reimbursement – has turned out much worse than the disease. Medicare's strategies for controlling costs by cutting reimbursement to physicians and hospitals continue to be ineffective. Hospitals have been able to dodge those cost-cutting bullets by adding procedural and acuity (disease severity) codes to increase their DRG reimbursements. Physicians have been successful in persuading Congress to waive the SGR multiple times; it would be unsustainable for them if put into full effect. Still, the "perverse incentives" in Medicare payments have continued to reward high-tech specialty procedures at the expense of primary care and face-to-face patient visits.

The hospital and physician communities have responded with a series of moves that have checkmated the country's ability to control costs. Essentially, through the mechanisms of low Medicare physician reimbursement for nonprocedural primary care and the hospital-based DRG system, the government has assured that it would pay hospitals and doctors poorly for certain patients and certain kinds of care. To remain solvent, the hospitals responded by taking care of the patients Medicare paid well for – and doing everything they could to generate as much income as possible from those patients to survive financially. Burdened with debt and increasing overhead, physicians responded by abandoning primary care and building out procedural facilities to perform high-tech care on their patients.

Oncology, for instance, is well reimbursed, so many communities now see expensive, Taj Mahal-style cancer centers being built in their midst. These capital-intensive expenditures clearly don't control overall healthcare costs; they're short-term, shortsighted tactics for hospitals and doctors to survive the current competitive environment. Physicians and hospital administrators are smart, and they're mastering the Medicare game. The government, after it loses one chess game and the next one starts, eventually catches on and changes tactics. But there are no Bobby Fischers working for Medicare. The government keeps changing the rules but losing the overall game, because they haven't identified the game's real goal: creating value in health care.

Physicians' siege mentality

A further complicating factor in the current healthcare crisis is the mindset of physicians today. When I talk to physicians around the country, they're frightened, they have extremely low morale right now, and they're stressed to the breaking point. Clearly, the constant ratcheting down of reimbursement and constant increase in the regulatory environment have forced physicians into a siege mentality.

When you're at war and sitting in a foxhole with artillery constantly coming in, you might be inclined to talk to your buddy next to you about Plato and the cave, what you think the real world ought to look like, and the future of medicine. But I suspect your primary focus is on keeping yourself together and staying alive. Most physicians today are working incredibly long hours, and while they may be surviving financially, they're not sure whether it will last – even for those physicians now doing well. They look around and see what's happened to other doctors who are leaving primary care, retiring early, or changing careers, and they're saying, "It's just a matter of time before that's me."

One of my cardiology colleagues recently shared those fears with me. I asked him why he works in the hospital until two in the morning every day of the week and never sees his wife or kids; even when he's not on call, he's in the hospital. He replied that he's paid well now, and doesn't know what's going to happen in the future. He's truly frightened, and that's what we're seeing throughout the physician community right now.

This siege mentality, to the detriment of everyone concerned, keeps physicians from getting more involved in the healthcare debate. When you have people who are chronically stressed and you introduce change, they're going to react negatively. Any change is stressful, even a positive change such as getting married or starting a new job. There's an especially stressed, negative, psychological dynamic and resistant mindset in the physician community right now. They're thinking, "The sky is falling, the shells are coming in. I don't care what you do, just don't put anything more on my plate right now; I don't have time for it."

This dynamic has pushed physicians into a reactive, almost victim mode, and it's a vicious cycle. Medicare makes another round of lowering their reimbursements and increasing the regulatory burden, and the hospital passes their regulatory requirements onto their physicians. The physicians react negatively; who doesn't when asked to work harder and earn less? Doctors haven't had time to step back, instead of reacting, and ask, "What could we do to prevent this problem, so we don't have to react and could instead play a more proactive leadership role in the healthcare crisis? What proposals could we put out there that would make sense?" None of the healthcare reform proposals on the table right now make sense from the physicians' perspective; and it makes sense that they don't make sense: They're all generated by nonclinicians.

Playing chess with docs

Playing chess with doctors is a losing proposition; they're always going to win. Even when the rules change, doctors quickly learn the new rules and adopt them to their advantage. When you cut reimbursement for primary care and reward expensive procedural specialists, what new phenomena do you see? Both new and long-practicing physicians are opting out of primary care. More and more medical graduates are selecting specialties that are procedure-based and therefore well compensated. Specialists are buying into ownership of surgical centers and diagnostic testing labs, and the overall utilization of high-tech, expensive procedures has skyrocketed.

Medicare has tried to intervene, but each success has been short-lived. The federal "Stark laws," for instance, which first went into effect in 2002 and apply to Medicare and other federally funded programs, prevent self-referrals from physicians in situations where doctors would benefit financially from the referral, such as doctors sending patients to an MRI facility the doctors themselves owned. Physicians were, however, still able to refer patients to a facility owned by a group practice, so the results of the Stark laws are limited. Government regulation has not been and will not be successful at controlling physician utilization so long as that utilization is reimbursed in a fee-for-service mode at a more favorable rate than primary care.

I often wonder what would have happened to overall healthcare costs, if years ago our society decided that every physician in the United States could make a guaranteed, comfortable living at a set amount so there would be no incentive to do more procedures. I doubt we'd be in the crisis we're in if there were no incentives for physicians to utilize more healthcare services, thereby costing more for both individual patients and the country's healthcare system at large.

In this hypothetical scenario, we as a society could have said to physicians, "If you admit more patients to the hospital, you don't make more money. If you do more surgeries or high-tech procedures, you don't make more money; and if you order more CT scans, you don't make more money. You only make money by spending time with patients." As a society, we might use some form of "relative value" in this hypothetical, deciding that if family doctors earn *x* dollars a year, for instance, then cardiologists should earn 1.5*x* and neurosurgeons should earn 2*x*. Whatever numbers might have ultimately been accepted, the point would have been to eliminate the unfair financial incentives in the system.

Is health care a commodity or an entitlement?

To sort through the complexity of the healthcare crisis, it's helpful to think of two arenas in terms of solutions. One arena holds the societal responsibility to more clearly define – perhaps redefine – health care in this country, a responsibility resolved through the political process and led by informed opinion. The second arena is the responsibility of the physician community. Regardless of how we decide as a society to define and fund health care, physician leaders are best poised to reduce cost within the system and generate real clinical value.

Physicians, healthcare executives, hospital administrators, payers, and others involved in healthcare delivery argue that health care is different from any other industry. While this is often used as an excuse to resist change, the argument does have validity; health care does pose unusually complex moral, financial, and social challenges.

First, we as a society have not defined what "health care" is. Some healthcare reform strategists would argue that health care is a commodity like any other and responds to pricing accordingly. Others would argue that health care is an entitlement, so that every citizen is entitled to receive health care regardless of his or her ability to pay. Two very different viewpoints – and in the final analysis, health care may not be either, but instead share elements of both.

Health care is not a free market, but some politicians talk about it as if it were. In a free market, no one stands between the buyer and the seller, or between the payer and the provider. If you walk into a Mercedes dealer with a Chevrolet budget, you aren't going to find a car you can afford, and the Mercedes dealer won't have any problem telling you to look elsewhere. That's a free market, but that's not health care.

It's hard to consider health care as a pure commodity, in part due to its multiple middlemen. The insurance company negotiates prices on behalf of the consumer; the physician directs patient referrals to hospitals. The medical director at a new emergency department, for instance, has to develop good relationships with the local emergency medical technicians (EMTs) – who direct patient referrals to the emergency department (ED) – so he's staying ahead of his competing ED a few miles away. Patients lying in the back of an ambulance are rarely in a position to choose which hospital they want to go to. Instead, the EMTs usually decide where they're taking patients, so the hospital's ED and nurses always have plenty of donuts and smiles on hand for them. Of course, if you're acutely ill and turn up in the emergency room, the ED staff will take care of you, even if you can't pay. In fact, this longstanding social contract was formally codified in the Emergency Treatment and Active Labor Act passed by the U.S. Congress in 1986, which specifically prohibits any other option.

On the other hand, if health care is an entitlement, then it raises the issue of who is responsible to choose the "right" service and to pay for it. Arguing that health care is a commodity puts the onus of responsibility on the consumer, whereas health care as an entitlement puts it on the government.

What do we as individuals owe society regarding health care, and what does society owe us? Should society provide the resources for everyone to have emergency care but not preventive care? For everyone to have preventive care, or only all children? Who owns the problem? Is it primarily a problem for individual consumers, for society at large, or a balance of the two? How do we as a country address these questions and decide what resources we're going to allocate for it? It's a debate worth having, because you can't solve a problem if you can't define it. Defining where health care fits along the entitlement-to-commodity continuum is a critical step in focusing the societal debate on reform.

What should health care include?

Our society has yet to agree collectively what "health care" includes, and because its scope hasn't been well defined, the public debate lacks focus, clarity, and momentum. Everyone would agree that if someone needs bypass surgery, that procedure falls in the realm of health care and should be eligible for health insurance benefits. At the other end of the spectrum, most people would agree that elective cosmetic surgery is not part of "essential" health care and should not be included in insured benefits.

But what about alternative health care like massage therapy, acupuncture, naturopathy, and herbal therapy? After years of intense lobbying by consumers and alternative healthcare providers, and despite the lack of scientifically proven benefit, these services are now included in many health insurance plans. Their inclusion has increased premiums for all. Should they be included in standard coverage paid by all subscribers, or should they be part of a "package-plus" benefit paid for by those who chose to – and can afford to – do so?

Once insurers decide to cover a given healthcare service, the utilization of that service increases immediately and often exponentially. Chiropractors are clearly excited to have chiropractic therapy covered by insurance policies; it increases their revenue and market share. Consumers are much more reluctant to go to massage therapists if they have to pay out-of-pocket for it. For consumers, their out-of-pocket costs for alternative medicine is a valid concern. Even more critical is that it's hard to get a handle on national healthcare expenses while consistently adding new services with unproven benefit and increasing their availability – another factor complicating an already complicated issue.

Who's paying?

Another issue is who's paying for health care? Who should? The bulk of most consumers' healthcare premiums are paid by someone else; it's a benefit paid by their employers or by the government through either Medicare or Medicaid. Even with the significant downturn in the U.S. economy in 2010, 59% of Americans under age 65 had employment-based insurance, and virtually all of those over age 65 had Medicare benefits, leaving 49 million people – 16% of the population – in America uninsured.

Only a small minority of people in this country today actually pays full cost out-of-pocket for their health care. While each year consumers are paying more for their health benefits through a higher percentage of increasing premiums, higher deductibles, and higher co-pays, the bulk of their healthcare costs remain indirect. Consumers' costs are covered by their employee benefits, paid for by direct wage reduction, or given as a government benefit paid through tax revenues. Shielding the consumer from experiencing the direct cost of health care has contributed to a moral hazard in which insurers, consumers, and providers can all drive up the use of medical services and contribute to inappropriate, inefficient expenditures responsible for much of the unsustainable rise in overall costs.

Health insurance: a prepaid benefit

Another complicating dynamic is medical insurance, which ties healthcare benefits to employment and works unlike any other kind of insurance. When you take your car in for routine maintenance, you don't use your car insurance; you pay for that out-of-pocket. In fact, even if you have an accident, it has to be a significant accident before, fearing significant rises in your premium, you report it to your insurance company and actually use your insurance. If you have disability insurance, you have a waiting period, and then you collect a percentage of your previous salary. Every type of insurance policy – except for health care – has significant disincentives for using it.

While the addition of co-pays has had some impact on overall healthcare costs without compromising the health of its beneficiaries, its impact is destined to be limited. The recent addition of Medicare Part D covering pharmaceutical costs to basic Medicare benefits is a good example of what happens when consumers no longer have to pay a significant portion of their healthcare costs out of their own pockets: Utilization of services rises and overall healthcare costs increase. The "commodity" becomes an "entitlement." Co-pays have been in place since the 1970s and are here to stay, but their overall impact on controlling national healthcare costs continues to be limited. Instead, as more benefits are added to the package, costs rise.

Lack of a value proposition

With so many medical services offered with little direct, transparent costs, few patients focus on value because it's not their own money they're spending. Without the push to define value, the healthcare crisis itself remains ill defined.

In most other arenas where money is spent, there's a clear concept of value: quality divided by cost. People who spend extra money on a car, who decide to buy a Mercedes instead of a Chevy, are doing so based on a value proposition, whether it's prestige, performance, reduced maintenance, or better resale value. You may disagree with them, but they understand the value proposition and are willing to part with their money because they see the value. They've done a calculation and determined that what they get for that money is worth it.

The dynamics of value propositions are likely to change over your lifetime. You might spend less money on a car as you get older because the value of status, for instance, may be lower than it is earlier in life. Whether evaluating the costs of a medical procedure such as putting in cardiac stents or a service such as expanding prescription drug coverage nationwide, the most rational approach will focus on value. The problem with health care is that we have not forced consumers, providers, or payers to define value. Because someone else is actually paying for most healthcare costs – employers, Medicare, or Medicaid – there's insufficient widespread concern and responsibility about overall costs, potentially creating an overly dependent society.

In health care, when you see your doctor and are told that you should have this test and then that procedure, you're likely to comply. Your insurance company may hassle you about covering all those tests but, despite the occasional horror story that makes the news, the overwhelming number of new and unproven procedures are quickly covered. Insurers can make it difficult, they can make you jump through hoops or make you pay a little extra, but the consumer usually wins. Resource utilization doesn't work like that in other industries: Health care is unique because the insured consumers aren't directly paying the bulk of their bill.

The point is that if you don't understand what's driving costs, you can't fix the costs. Nurses' salaries are not killing us; physicians' salaries are not killing us. Physician utilization is what's doing us in. What's killing us is that Dr. Lean can take care of a patient with congestive heart failure and do a really good job at *x* dollars; and Dr. Chubb takes care of the same kind of patient and spends 20*x* – with no better results. Overutilization hasn't been the focus of the current healthcare debate – but it needs to be, and it would be if doctors were more involved and taking leadership roles in healthcare reform. Even the minority of politicians and policy makers who are focusing on cost can't fix it, because as a country we're still essentially paying piecemeal with fee-for-service, and docs with political clout are wed to that kind of reimbursement and can't yet see the upside of changing it.

Financial conflicts between doctors and hospitals

Consider again that simple operational example that a hospital can't bill Medicare until a discharge summary has been dictated. But physicians have no incentive to dictate discharge summaries and verify their accuracy when patients leave the hospital, and they're too busy to donate any of their time. Their incentive is to return to their offices as fast as possible where they're going to make some money seeing patients, or get into the cath lab or the OR to do some procedures. Physicians don't get paid to dictate discharge summaries or to approve their accuracy after they've been transcribed, and they certainly don't get paid more to do it in a timely manner, when the hospital wishes it were done.

At this moment, hundreds of undictated discharge summaries sit in every hospital's record room, waiting for physicians to dictate and then review. You can imagine the cost to the hospital when they have millions of dollars' worth of revenue they can't bill for, sitting in the record room, waiting for physicians to dictate. At one hospital, for instance, a project by a healthcare consulting group used a system known as "Lean Healthcare," a set of operational and organizational tools adapted from the "lean" management style popularized by Toyota, which saved the hospital $1.5 million a year in payroll-related costs and reversed 10% of the hospital's $1 million in negative cash flow due to medical record delinquency.

The regulatory environment driven by the Joint Commission has made that situation enormously worse by requiring that hospitals now provide a "medication reconciliation" for every patient to make sure that all of a patient's drugs reconcile at discharge. Many patients come in with multiple drugs, they go home with other drugs, and they're not necessarily the same; or they are the same but have different names and dosing. It's difficult on the patients. Now, in addition to dictating discharge summaries, physicians have been charged by hospitals to perform a drug reconciliation prior to every patient discharge, another time-consuming task doctors don't get paid for. The intention is good; otherwise, patients leave the hospital thoroughly confused about what medications they're supposed to take and how. The effect of mandatory drug reconciliation, however, creates another responsibility the hospital has to assume without the authority for implementation, which resides in the control of its physician staff.

The bottom line is that the relationship between physicians and hospitals is complex; they're partners, and yet they're competitors. They have some areas in which their interests may overlap, but in many areas their interests conflict – such as with hospitalization. The financial reality is that hospitals want the patient in and out of the hospital as fast as possible with the lowest utilization of in-house resources. The hospital has to pay for every resource a doctor uses, and given the DRG system, the hospital will only receive a certain amount of money no matter how many resources the doctor uses in caring for a given patient.

But for doctors, the more care they provide while patients are in the hospital, the better, because they're billing for everything they do. There's no urgency toward discharge from the doctors' point of view since their fees aren't prospectively determined. To get the patient out of the hospital means a doctor needs to see the patient more often, needs to be on the phone more often to be aware of what's going on with labs or diagnostic tests, and needs to be sure that he or she completes the discharge summary and drug reconciliation as soon as possible. Even free-agent hospitalists who work in a hospital bill in the fee-for-service scheme; or, if they're employed by a hospital or group practice, their employer is billing their services out as fee-for-service. So doctors have to ask themselves, "Am I going to spend my time dictating discharge summaries and doing drug reconciliations for the hospital, which take up my unpaid time, or see four or five patients in the same amount of time, knowing I'd get paid for all of those patient encounters?"

The new salaried physicians: an incomplete strategy

One of the recent strategies by hospitals to control costs, beginning in the 1990s, was to employ physicians on salary, by hiring individual doctors and acquiring group practices. According to *The New England Journal of Medicine* in May 2011, more than half of all practicing physicians were then employed by hospitals or integrated delivery systems. But that tactic alone doesn't address overutilization of hospital resources by physicians, because their salaries embrace the same incentives doctors had when billing privately.

Most salaried physicians still work on a fee-for-service basis, what's also called a "production basis," which drives how they get paid. The hospital essentially collects their billings and then writes them a check, so the financial incentives for physicians haven't changed much, even though they're salaried. Salaried physicians still work within a fee-for-service system in terms of how they get paid and incentivized by hospitals, as well as how hospitals get paid by private insurance and Medicare. Putting physicians on salary often simply shifts who's doing the billing paperwork.

At one large, successful hospital in Seattle, for instance, all physicians are salaried, and the hospital contracts with several insurers, including Medicare. When the hospital bills Medicare for a cardiology procedure, a cardiac catheterization done by Dr. Chubb and one done by Dr. Lean is reimbursed at the same rate back to the hospital. The hospital leadership can incentivize doctors any way they choose, but at this point, since the employer-hospital increases its revenue by increasing salaried physician billings, the compensation mechanism for cardiologists and procedure-driven, surgery-driven specialists is a salary base, plus a "productivity-oriented" bonus depending on how many procedures they do. Most hospitals aren't incentivizing based on efficiency, because Dr. Chubb's overutilization of hospital-based resources likely increases his fee-for-service reimbursement and therefore increases hospital revenue. Conversely, Dr. Lean, who is four times as efficient in patient care with the same or better patient outcomes, may produce lower fee-for-service billings.

New physician incentives: value

How likely is it that hospitals would start incentivizing physicians on efficiency or value rather than on number of procedures? It would happen about ten milliseconds after the reimbursement system changed to reward efficiency and value. That kind of change would have to be driven by the economics of a new reimbursement structure, because hospital CEOs would have trouble keeping their jobs if their hospitals didn't remain financially viable.

This isn't cynicism; it's pragmatism. The vast majority of doctors has morals and wants to provide good patient care, and they have enough intelligence to pursue other careers to make a lot more money if they were primarily interested in money. A doctor who gets into Harvard Medical School could probably get into Harvard Business School. But physicians have families, mortgages, and medical school debts, and they're going to have to survive financially in the future. The same holds true for hospitals; they're going to have to survive. Hospital CEOs want to do the right thing, but if they're not profitable, they're not feeding the coffers, and that's still a motivating force – even for charity hospitals. Catholic healthcare systems clearly have a mission – to take care of low-income people – and they would argue that their profits help them do just that. If they don't have the money to spend, they can't subsidize care for the people who need it.

Clearly, physicians have been put in a bind over the last 20 years, due to how much health care has changed and the crunch it has put on doctors. What they thought they would be doing when they started practicing medicine differs widely from how they're actually spending their time – on legal, financial, and administrative paperwork. It seems that medicine is becoming less about the ideals that inspired doctors to go into medicine in the first place.

That's why we need a system that guarantees physicians adequate reimbursement without perverse financial incentives. The actual dollar amount wouldn't matter as much to many physicians, at this point, as a sense of long-term security. If neurosurgeons are making half a million dollars a year, that might sound like a lot of money, but we as a society may decide they're worth that, given the complicated surgeries they're able to do. But whatever the number is, let's spend the money

– incentivize doctors – to take care of patients, to be able to spend time with them and time with their families, to map out the most efficient protocols for various medical problems, and to use technology in a more thoughtful, measured way.

Physicians, not bureaucrats, need to be the ones asking the tough questions – is this technology really necessary, is it really going to help, or is it unnecessary? – with the financial incentives for using that technology taken completely out of the picture. It's not that technology shouldn't be used, but used more wisely. Take the financial incentives away to overuse high-tech diagnostic and therapeutic procedures, and physicians won't be driven or even tempted. They'd know they won't make any more money to use technology more often, and they won't be incentivized to go out and buy the latest new technology to support and market their practices. Ultimately, most doctors would be a lot happier with that. A few doctors really are born entrepreneurs, but the majority simply wants to take care of patients and has felt forced to become entrepreneurial just to keep up.

An integrated system to control costs

Who knows how to produce value in health care? Clinicians. No one else has the scientific education and clinical training to do it. Cardiologists, for example, are the only people who can intelligently reevaluate current cardiac care and protocols to ask, "What's happening now in the way we look at cardiology patients, from the moment they come in our offices until the day they die? What are we doing that we don't need to do, and what aren't we doing that we ought to do? From a quality and value perspective, what is the best way to care for these patients?" Not enough healthcare policy makers – and certainly not enough physicians – are having these conversations.

There's an incredible amount of waste in medicine. We're doing routine EKGs that are worthless, treadmill tests that have no predictive value – and the list goes on. Physicians spend too much of their time doing paperwork from Medicare, private insurers, the hospital where they practice, and regulatory agencies – much of which someone else could be doing for a physician's review, or perhaps doesn't have to be done at all because it adds no real value to the healthcare system.

If we said to hospitals and physicians, "Here's one check to take care of a certain population of patients; it's all you get, figure it out," they'd figure it out in a heartbeat. The Accountable Care Organizations proposed in the Affordable Care Act mandate this with a top-down approach, where bureaucrats would determine acceptable "outcomes," decide which players in health care win and which lose, who's paid more and who's paid less. A smarter alternative would give integrated delivery systems the same reimbursement and the same expected minimal outcomes, and let the market decide which of them wins and loses.

I'm not suggesting that we adopt the Canadian system, but I am suggesting that American physicians play a central leadership role in salvaging what's best about our healthcare system, while helping to control costs and develop local efforts to create value in health care. In the future, Medicare may start bundling payment for more services, such as paying not only for the hospitalization for a diagnosis of congestive heart failure but for all costs, including all physician fees, in one prospective payment. Medicare may later decide to extend that one-time payment scheme to both hospitalization and 30-day post-hospitalization costs; or it may even eventually start paying a one-time prospective payment for a year's worth of services for an enrollee's care, a flat "global payment" scheme similar to those explored by Massachusetts, a leader in state healthcare reform, to control healthcare costs. As *The New York Times* reported in October 2011, Blue Cross Blue Shield of Massachusetts has used global payments successfully since 2009, when it began paying groups of doctors and hospitals flat fees to care for over 600,000 patients cooperatively.

But because physicians rather than bureaucrats have the required medical expertise, physicians should take the lead on disease management, evaluate patient populations and demographics, and get involved on multiple strategic levels to understand what the systemic challenges are and how to devise a sensible proposal, based on value, for meaningful national healthcare reform. Instead of reacting to proposals coming from people who don't fully understand health care, why don't we as physicians lead the process, work with the various stakeholders, and say, "Here are the ideal outcomes for patients with heart failure. Here's what we know absolutely works; here's what we know absolutely does not work; here's where we're not sure. Let's develop a protocol we can all work with to reduce costs while keeping the quality of our patient care high." These protocols would be designed to work across the healthcare delivery spectrum, whether patients are still employed, at home, or in a hospital or long-term care facility. The protocols would include patients and family members in decision-making and cover what they can do with self-care and the latest behavioral medicine strategies for adopting healthy lifestyles.

There are untold patient-care improvements and cost-saving measures that physicians haven't had time to think about because they've been too busy reacting to changes initiated by Medicare, Medicaid, hospitals, and regulatory agencies. The current healthcare system continues to force doctors to react. Practicing physicians have little leeway or incentive to think about the healthcare system as a whole. In fact, many have been disincentivized to think proactively about these issues at all.

Training physicians to think proactively

A key new role for physicians would be setting up detailed, cost-effective protocols and systems to track patients more consistently along a continuum of care, instead of the current episodic care, with its "we'll-see-you-in-a-month" approach. But physicians have traditionally never been involved in conversations to strategize cost-effective care together with other stakeholders on a system-wide level. That's not what we've been reimbursed to do.

Physicians don't need to be given incentives to provide better patient care if they're in an integrated system with a long-term, system-wide mindset, because the vast majority of doctors already have that moral incentive hard-wired into their psyches via their training. But physicians who are now being forced to focus on their incomes do need to be given new incentives to focus on patient care. As a society, we need to make them secure enough financially, without having to rely on perverse incentives to know that they won't go under if they spend time thinking about how to improve patient care and control unnecessary costs. If physicians didn't have so many financial pressures and were adequately reimbursed for spending time thinking about clinical protocols and working on systems, they'd be a lot more willing to allocate a portion of patient care to other kinds of providers, such as nurse practitioners – at considerably less cost to the national system.

Right now physicians are competing for their piece of the national healthcare budget with other providers: hospitals, nurses, physicians' assistants, nurse practitioners, acupuncturists, chiropractors, naturopaths, and others. When a physician writes an order for home care visits and Medicare pays for them, it's another incentive for Medicare to reduce physician reimbursement through the "sustained growth rate" cuts, since it can then appear that the need for physician services has dropped.

But if you're in a system where all levels of providers receive a single prospective payment check for patient care, the nurse going out to provide care in patients' homes is saving money that could augment physician reimbursement and patient access. In this new kind of integrated system it might not even be a nurse; it could be a home health aide. Extending care into homes, working systematically across the entire continuum of care, could save money while maintaining quality of care. Today's fragmented reimbursement scheme, pitting providers against one another, can't support comprehensive care. But with healthcare integration, we as providers would be asking ourselves, "Is this person or process adding value or not?"

In my years of clinical practice as a cardiologist, I saw multiple, major issues with the delivery of care, where physician-directed pathways would have been extremely valuable in assuring that care was beneficial as well as cost-effective. But many physicians have never really seen themselves in that strategic role. Leaving the daily pressures of clinical practice has allowed physicians like me to step back and look at the big picture, to assess what's working and not working from a broader, system-wide perspective. Given the urgency of the current healthcare crisis and all that has to happen to turn it around, if we as physicians abdicate those visioning, planning, and decision-making roles to someone else, it's going to be done without the clinical expertise and experience needed to set medical priorities and design the best protocols and practices for the country as a whole. That's where physicians need to be today: leading the effort toward reforming health care.

What's not driving costs: "fraud and abuse"

"Medicare fraud and abuse" is a media sound bite distortion; it's not a common problem, just a media-sexy one. People love to read stories such as the one mentioned previously about the Baltimore area cardiologist and tell themselves a comforting story: There's no real problem with the system, just a problem with the few who are abusing the system. True, the actions of the Baltimore area cardiologist and the hospital that recruited him can be categorized as "Medicare fraud and abuse," and the elimination of this kind of egregious behavior will reduce Medicare costs. But which is more costly to the U.S. taxpayer: this outlier case, or perpetuating a system that hides its true costs from the public and rewards overutilization of unnecessary procedures, while at the same time penalizing physicians who spend time consulting with patients and answering their questions? Who is more fraudulent: the physician who abuses stent placement or the politicians who tell their constituents that they can have unlimited access to health care and have someone else pay for it? The hospital that recruits specialists to increase their volume of expensive, profitable procedures or the spin doctors who invent so-called "death panels" and claim they're in the health reform laws as a way to steer consumers away from reform?

There's nowhere near enough "Medicare fraud and abuse" by physicians and hospitals to pay for the extra entitlements that some members of Congress keep asking for. The logical conclusion is that too many political leaders never read the entire, lengthy, healthcare reform proposal of 2010 – or simply don't yet fully understand the intricacies of how clinical medicine and health care actually work.

To practice safe, value-driven medicine, physicians don't need bureaucrats looking over their every move. Bureaucrats create rules they think will lead to better outcomes and then need to create more rules each year to justify their paychecks. "Medicare fraud and abuse" is a prime example of this, but the fundamental factor that defines true fraud and abuse is intent. There's no question that a large number of billing errors are made accidentally each year, given the increasingly complicated, ever-changing medical coding involved in today's billing. If a billing code is incorrect, however, it doesn't necessarily mean anyone had an "intent" to deceive Medicare. From a national perspective, imagine the system-wide algorithms and the dollars spent on "fraud and abuse," with an army of bureaucrats monitoring, consultants giving advice and planning tactics, and specialized medical coders employed for compliance assurance.

It's not a sensible reform strategy for three reasons. If we paid providers prospectively to care for certain groups of patients, there wouldn't be fraud and abuse because providers would be managing their own budgets. Also, increasing regulation adds funding to the healthcare budget that goes to bureaucrats rather than to healthcare providers where it's sorely needed. Finally, the reality is that "fraud and abuse" numbers are all only estimates. When a politician says, "We can save millions of dollars by eliminating "Medicare fraud and abuse," that number comes from a faulty definition of fraud and abuse. If a physician bills Medicare for a code and uses the wrong diagnostic code, that could simply be a doctor who's been up for 48 hours and wrote a "0" by mistake instead of a "1," or a doctor who hasn't updated his billing system based on the most recent Medicare changes. Screening all billing errors for "fraud and abuse" is inflammatory, derogatory to physicians, and worse – it's misleading to the American public to imply that there's that much fraud and abuse actually happening.

How are we going to uncover those few cases of real fraud and abuse? In 2008, there were 661,400 doctors practicing in the United States. A few, no doubt, were practicing fraud and abuse, given the bell-shape moral curve of any group of people. But the government proposes putting even more required forms in place to ensure that all physicians aren't doing something wrong, which would require hiring people to make sure all those forms are collected, reviewing all those forms, and then if a questionable form turns up, hiring people to go back into suspect physicians' offices, shut them down for a few days, and look through all of their charts to make sure that they weren't seeing the tip of the iceberg.

Will increased bureaucratic policing save healthcare dollars? No. Will it further demoralize physicians? Count on it. It doesn't make any sense, but eliminating fraud and abuse continues to be touted as a major solution to the healthcare crisis, though the issue is never fully explained to the public. When the nonpartisan Congressional Budget Office (CBO) reviewed the 2010 health reform legislation proposal and asked the obvious question – "How are we going to pay for all this?" – the answer can't be only to eliminate "fraud and abuse." In fact, the conclusion of the CBO's Congressional testimony in July 1995 stated, "Fraud and abuse clearly exist in Medicare, just as in all other public and private health plans, but estimates of potential losses from fraud and abuse are inherently speculative. If HCFA (the Health Care Financing Administration) and private insurers had good information about the extent of the problem, they would know how to eliminate it." CBO testimony further stated that "the amount of savings to be expected is uncertain because diminishing returns are sure to set in as additional resources are devoted to those activities."

The proposed cost savings from "fraud and abuse" has been a ridiculously large number: $50 billion. That number only makes sense if you decide that every time someone miscodes something, even accidentally within the constant revisions of the codes, that's "fraud and abuse." When you have far-reaching issues that are as complex as health care, the easiest way for politicians to deal with them is to throw out sound bites, just as the Republicans did with their ads about "death squads" during the Clinton era, with the characters of "Harry and Louise" terrified that the Democrats would take all health care away. Health care is too complicated to be explained or understood by sound bites.

The bottom line? All these minor tinkerings with a broken, unsustainable healthcare system are an attempt to avoid the hugely difficult political decisions that would have to be made, by politicians and the country as a whole, to solve the crisis long-term. Talking about fraud and abuse is politically safe because everyone can agree, "Let's not allow fraud and abuse." It's like saying you're "pro peace." Everyone is "pro peace." The argument isn't about whether you want peace; it's about how you arrive at that goal.

CHAPTER 2
What's Really Driving Costs?

American health care has increasingly become a financial rat's nest, with a number of different historical threads from multiple industries interlocking into hugely knotty issues over the years. The current healthcare crisis also raises essential societal questions about what health care should be in our country and who deserves what, both as consumers receiving care and as medical professionals reimbursed for providing care. Resolving the healthcare crisis requires an understanding of how the system has evolved over the past to become the behemoth it is today. The number of issues at stake and the different stakeholders affected by the healthcare crisis are phenomenally diverse; arguably, no other domestic issue today is quite so far-reaching or complex.

The role of insurance

Health insurance is a relatively new phenomenon. In the early 1950s, in the days before health insurance as an industry took hold, Americans paid for their health care out of pocket. A few charity hospitals were formed, often along religious lines, such as the Catholic healthcare systems supported by charitable foundations and donations, where patients could apply for a sliding scale when they were admitted to the hospital. Otherwise, patients went to a private hospital and paid whatever the hospital claimed their care cost, whether it was a small rural hospital in Montana or a ritzy city hospital in Manhattan. In the preinsurance model of American health care, patients were financially responsible for all of the care they received and paid hospitals and doctors directly for whatever care they were given. When it came to physician payment for both inpatient care in the hospital and outpatient care in physicians' offices, doctors and patients essentially negotiated among themselves.

At that time, before the 1950s, most physicians were what we'd call "lower-middle-class" today; they earned professional wages but certainly weren't wealthy. In small towns, doctors bartered with patients: They'd set a broken leg or stitch up a cut and the patient might pay in cash – or might deliver a cord of wood to the doctor's house.

Beginning in the early 1950s, the growth in the number of U.S. businesses drove employers to find new ways to woo employees to work for them, and the idea of health insurance was born – that you could buy medical insurance to pay for medical bills. Large, successful companies like Westinghouse, GE, and GM began offering health insurance as an employee benefit, and soon thereafter the unions started using medical coverage as a key strategic leverage point in wage and benefit negotiations. Like most benefits, it eventually became an "entitlement" in Americans' minds, a social expectation that working for a company or the government meant receiving health insurance benefits.

It's fascinating to compare our country's healthcare spending before and after health insurance began. When health insurance first started, we were spending about 1% of GDP on health care. That number saw a gradual rise until about 1965, when Medicare was started, and then healthcare costs began to explode; we're spending nearly 18% of GDP now. That's partly why insurers try to "cherry pick" the healthiest customers. When Medicare began offering different plans and letting private insurers sell and administer those plans, it hoped that initiating market competition among different Medicare plans would save Medicare money. One insurer advertised for enrollees solely in fitness clubs – the ultimate "cherry-picking" strategy to find the healthiest clients so they could spend the least money paying for their medical care.

Today's physicians may recognize the flawed thinking behind health insurance plans and policies; it's part of the morale problem as a profession. But because they're all fighting for their own turf and their own survival, physicians aren't getting involved with the healthcare crisis, and many don't fully recognize how fast and far downhill the current system's going.

The fee-for-service windfall

As Paul Starr, Princeton professor and author, so richly detailed in his Pulitzer-prize-winning book, *The Social Transformation of American Health Care*, organized medicine – both doctors and hospitals – fought Medicare. They didn't want the government to get involved; they didn't want what they perceived to be socialized medicine. The irony is that when you look at what actually happened, Medicare made many doctors and hospitals quite wealthy.

Perhaps unknowingly when they designed Medicare, the government didn't change the fee-for-service mentality or reimbursement system. Back when you as a consumer were bartering or paying out of pocket, the fee-for-service system made sense. The doctor told you how much a treatment would cost, and you'd decide whether or not you wanted it – or could afford it. Clearly, you're not going to spend money on something that you don't see as valuable and necessary, or can't afford even if it is necessary. You might be just barely scratching out a living, and decide that you'll take your chances and not have treatment.

From a social standpoint, the old fee-for-service system had ethical issues – the rich could afford health care, the poor couldn't – although the system worked from a purely economic exchange standpoint: one buyer, one seller, a negotiated price. When insurance companies came in, they simply became the middlemen between providers and patients and kept the fee-for-service model for a long time. The insurers wanted to pay doctors through their insurance plan, so they asked doctors, "How do we do this? How do we pay you?" Doctors responded by telling the insurers what they charged for each of their various procedures. Essentially, doctors set their own rates, which became what were then called "usual and customary fees." Insurers basically agreed to pay whatever doctors told them treatment cost. Every few years, as inflation and overhead costs rose, hospitals and physicians calculated a cost-of-living increase and passed it on to insurance companies as their new "usual and customary fees," and the insurers agreed. Today's physicians' fees are based on previous years' insurer-doctor contracts with "adjustments."

So physicians who were charging $10 for an office visit in their community when their patients couldn't afford to pay more out-of-pocket could now charge $30, $40, $50 – whatever the insurance companies would pay. Insurance was a huge financial boon to both doctors and hospitals, and not only due to the increase in fees they were paid. The insurers also paid consistently within a few weeks of billing, so it reduced the "bad debt" problem for both hospitals and physicians, from patients who either couldn't or wouldn't pay. So despite all the loud objections of organized medicine, it was a bonanza. Of course, adding a new layer of administrators – insurance companies – added a new layer of costs to our country's healthcare system as a whole.

Curiously, as it turns out, the naysayers were right. Back in the 1950s, the American Medical Association feared that letting insurers or the government start paying for medical care meant that they would have tremendous control over physicians and that there could come a day when payers would push back and say, "We're not paying for that treatment," or "We're now going to change the way we pay." But in fact both physicians and hospitals benefited for a long time.

One of the issues now with cost for private insurers and government is to convince others that it's perfectly appropriate for those paying the bills to start looking at what they're getting for their money.

Surprisingly, it wasn't until the 1980s that payers, both private insurers and government-sponsored programs, started looking at the growth of healthcare spending compared to GDP, and asked, "Why are we spending so much more than every other developed country in health care? Is this really necessary? Is it sustainable? What can we do to limit it?" But from the beginning of Medicare in 1965 until the 1980s, the third-party-payer system, with insurance companies and Medicare footing the bill, was a windfall for providers.

Insurers: funder of medical innovation

Here's the rub. We as a society also benefited – hugely – from that windfall. Since the late 1960s, the United States has led the world in medical innovation through an explosive growth in technology, drugs, devices, and diagnostic imaging, such as imaging techniques that reduce the need for invasive diagnostic procedures; medical devices and drugs that prolong life in a variety of cardiac conditions and save lives during heart attacks; vaccinations against a host of life-threatening diseases; antibiotics that significantly reduce disease mortality; new drugs to treat disease and limit the need for surgical intervention; and a host of new classes of medications that stop debilitating migraine headaches, treat depression, reduce the severity of arthritis, regulate the immune system to make lifesaving organ transplantation possible, and countless more.

These major advances were funded in large part because medical device and drug companies knew they could set prices that would be reimbursed by private insurance companies and Medicare. If these companies could identify a large enough market, knowing that most of that market had access to private insurance or Medicare, they had a good cushion for investment. While many of these procedures helped patients by providing needed care, they also drove up national spending. The National Center for Health Statistics, for example, reports that knee replacements rose by 40% between 2000 and 2004 – and expects that procedure to grow by a whopping 673% by 2030, thanks in large part to the aging and active baby boomer generation.

This new landscape appears vastly different from the 1950s. Back then, you might identify a great new drug, but you knew that it would cost millions to develop through expensive medical technology, and you could only charge a limited amount to private-pay patients for the drug. A dollar a pill? Back in the 1950s, no one would pay a dollar a pill if they had to pay out-of-pocket. Today, while wildly expensive drugs grab the headlines, the more common medications clearly illustrate the impact of insurance coverage. If a Medicare patient with cardiovascular disease without Medicare Part D, prescription drug coverage, went to a Walgreen's pharmacy in Seattle this year for a few relatively inexpensive, generic medications, his or her monthly out-of-pocket costs (retail pharmacy price plus co-pays) would be significantly higher than if that same patient had prescription drug coverage with Medicare.

***Without* Medicare Part D**	
Simvastatin 20 mg $28.99 + $2.60 co-pay	$31.95
Lisinopril 20 mg $20.79 + $2.60 co-pay	$23.39
Spironolactone 50 mg $45.99 + $2.60 co-pay	$48.59
Amiodarone 200 mg $106.98 + $2.60 co-pay	$109.50
Carvedilol 12.5 mg $21.99 + $2.60 co-pay	$24.59
Total monthly out-of-pocket costs without Medicare Part D	$238.02

***With* Medicare Part D**	
Monthly premium	$30.00
Monthly portion of yearly deductible	$26.83
Co-pay of $2.60 x 5 above drugs	$13.00
Total monthly out-of-pocket costs with Medicare Part D	$69.83

With Medicare Part D, this hypothetical patient needing comparatively modest drugs pays less than one-third (29%) of the monthly cost compared to patients without that coverage. You see the complexity: While it's socially responsible that an estimated 29 million Americans in 2011 were covered by Medicare Part D drug benefits, according to Reuters, it also costs our country's healthcare system a considerable amount of money, which takes a big bite out of overall funding for other services. Again, the point is to understand and compare the value of various forms of medical care, coverage, and services.

The growth of the pharmaceutical and medical device industries rubs both ways. Some of the new drugs and technologies are truly magical, so our health as a society has benefited tremendously from the last 50 years of medical innovation. Another benefit: If you look at the U.S. economy today, the well-paying jobs that offer growth, outside of specialized high-tech companies, are in health care. Healthcare professionals dominate the top-paying industries in America, according to the federal Bureau of Labor Statistics, which noted in its annual report in 2010 that nine of the 10 highest-paid jobs came from the healthcare industry; corporate executives were the only other group that made the Top 10. That same year, health care was responsible for 30% to 45% of viable new job creation in the United States.

In the future, if we start to rein in costs as a country, then we have to accept that controlling costs means that healthcare research, technology, and employment will all take a hit. The upside of controlling costs is that we'll be better able to compete in the global economy, but the downside may be fewer healthcare jobs or the same number of jobs that pay lower salaries. We'll also have to figure out who's going to fund the next round of innovations. Some smaller medical device or pharmaceutical companies will likely go under, and big companies may scale back on their research because they don't know what their return on investment will be.

The United States has been leading the world in developing medical technology because this is where the money is. Innovation isn't happening as much in Europe; in European countries, the government sets and enforces prices for healthcare services and procedures. The overwhelming majority of Europeans is covered by national healthcare systems, where there's a limit on what physicians can charge per procedure, such as per stent, or on the number of stents they can put in patients per year.

That's also what happens in Canada. If a patient needs an elective stent in Canada, they're up against the reality of the Canadian healthcare budget, and if that year's budget has run out, the patient waits until the next year. When you look at stent utilization, open heart surgery, or any other high-tech procedure and compare per capita rates, the United States' use of that technology is much higher than in other countries.

In fact, medical innovators who develop technology in their home countries often end up coming to the United States, which results in more rapid development of the technology and attracts an increasingly medically sophisticated "brain pool." One of the early developers of intracoronary stenting, for instance, Andreas Gruentzig, performed the first coronary balloon angioplasty in 1977 in a private institute in Zurich, and in 1980 came to Emory University in Atlanta, Georgia, because that's where the money was to continue his research.

Clearly, the positive side to insurance has also included increased access to care for Americans who would otherwise not be able to afford the surgeries, medications, and other medical services they need. With insurance, because there is limited financial penalty, some people access the healthcare system for prevention and early symptoms of disease, rather than wait until catastrophic illness to seek care. So health insurance has had a complex, nuanced history in our country with a blend of pros and cons.

Perverse incentives drive overutilization

The Organisation for Economic Co-operation and Development (OECD) compares the use of MRI and CT among its member countries.

Data from 2010 shows that while the average developed country in the OECD performs 139 CT scans per thousand citizens, the United States performs 228 per thousand. The average number of MRI scans is 49 per thousand people; in the United States it's 91 – nearly twice as many. Why? Because our fee-for-service reimbursement scheme creates built-in, "perverse incentives" for certain kinds of care, and "healthy reimbursement numbers" for the doctor and hospital don't necessarily correlate with the most effective, high-value care.

Public and private insurance have greatly impacted not only overall costs but also how fees are structured and paid. When physicians perform procedures in their private-practice offices, they can charge a "technical fee" in addition to their "professional fee," or "pro fee." The professional fee pays for the physician's time, and the technical fee pays for the technology, including amortizing its capital expense and interest over time. Because the technical fee is much higher than the professional fee, it creates a financial incentive for physicians and hospitals to own their own diagnostic equipment and perhaps do more diagnostic testing than is necessary for quality care. A physician who reads an MRI, for instance, might be paid $60 for the professional fee to do the interpretation, but might receive $1,000 or even more from the insurers for the "technical component" of providing the MRI.

A more recent component of healthcare billing is the "facility fee," which has driven the phenomenon of hospitals creating specialty clinics as part of their facilities. When hospitals purchase physicians' practices and move them from private-practice offices onto the hospital campus, they're allowed, in essence, to charge patients a double co-pay. Move a pulmonologist into a hospital-based Pulmonary Care Center, for instance, and the hospital can charge an extra co-pay for each patient visit, currently from $20 to $50, depending on the patient's insurance plan. One co-pay covers the professional fees to pay the pulmonologist and the second co-pay covers facility fees to pay for the costs of providing the facility and equipment, including the technical component.

Sample Bill: Abdominal MRI	
Total patient responsibility	$3,012.30
Patient's responsibility for Facility Fee	$2,645.30
Patient's responsibility for Professional Fee	$367.00

Unfortunately for consumers, the facility fee they have to pay to the hospital or clinic where a procedure is performed shows up as a second co-pay – one for the facility fee and one for the professional fee that's paid to the treating physician. The extra costs of the dual co-pay, especially for patients on fixed incomes, can inhibit them from seeking routine care or even exclude them from care entirely if they can no longer afford to pay twice as much to see the specialist they used to see when his practice wasn't part of a hospital facility.

From a larger perspective, these dual co-pays clearly drive up overall healthcare costs, both for the individual patient and the country as a whole. If a hospital buys a cardiology group practice, for instance, and moves them onto its campus, the hospital can increase their revenue by charging a facility fee every time a patient comes to see the cardiologist, even if it's simply for an office visit.

In addition, in the physicians' minds, because Medicare keeps cutting their fees for outpatient office visits, becoming an employee for a hospital brings the potential for new financial incentives. Some physicians' fees are higher when they perform their procedures in a hospital setting versus in a private-practice office. Medicare's current reimbursement scheme, in fact, encourages doctors to perform procedures in a hospital-owned facility because they can earn much more money. If a cardiologist's professional fee for a typical procedure is *x* dollars, the additional technical fee earned for that procedure may be as much as 50% higher if performed in a hospital-owned facility versus in a private-practice outpatient office. For other procedures, the professional fee might be only 10% to 33% of the technical fee. The reality is that Medicare reimburses a physician more for a cardiac catheterization procedure if the hospital-employed physician works for a hospital that owns the cath lab where the procedure is done, creating further incentives that drive up utilization.

"Chronic remunerative medicine"

From the cardiologists' perspective, there are a lot of unknowns and unproven variables in how we practice cardiology. We do routine EKGs, and if someone has surgery, we typically do follow-up stress testing, in some cases as often as every six months. But in fact, if patients aren't symptomatic, no data suggests that we should be doing anything other than treating them with statins (lipid-lowering agents) and aspirin, so why are we doing these other tests? What's the value of ordering an EKG every three months for a patient when cardiologists don't agree on how often EKGs should be done, and in fact there's little evidence that they need to be done at all? Who's actually benefiting? Furthermore, how often do we really need to monitor patients' blood chemistries if they're on a statin? Some doctors check blood chemistries only if patients are symptomatic. Doctors who own their own labs often order muscle enzyme testing much more frequently.

Implanting cardiac stents in patients suffering from a heart attack saves lives and preserves heart muscle – an undeniable advance for patients. In practice, however, most stents are implanted in patients who aren't having heart attacks. The data is clear: Stents work no better than medications in prolonging life and reducing new heart attack risk in patients who undergo elective stent procedures. It's a good argument for integrated care. If interventional cardiologists were part of a group of physicians managing one shared fund for all patient care, they'd be much more circumspect about what they were doing in the cath lab with cardiac procedures.

There's a phenomenon called "chronic remunerative medicine," in which patients essentially become an annuity for the unscrupulous physician. Patients don't have the medical training to know whether a procedure is truly necessary or when a physician may be overutilizing care.

Let's be clear: The vast majority of physicians are ethical professionals who don't intend to do this, but the system needs only a few who practice chronic remunerative medicine to create incredible problems with overutilization. It's not unique to cardiology, of course, but can play out in any specialty where patients have ongoing, lifelong medical conditions associated with tests and procedures that are well reimbursed by Medicare and private insurers.

How hospitals play chess with the Feds

About 10 years ago, Medicare analysts decided that outpatient medicine was less expensive than inpatient medicine, so Medicare would start paying a little bit more for a procedure if it was performed as an outpatient procedure, as a financial incentive to keep patients out of hospitals and in doctors' offices instead. Suddenly every cardiologist wanted to own a cardiac catheterization lab to perform outpatient procedures to diagnose and treat coronary artery disease, an echocardiogram machine to do ultrasound testing, and a nuclear camera for noninvasive evaluation of heart perfusion and function. Cardiologists bought these relatively expensive pieces of equipment because their return on investment looked so good.

In 2010, when Medicare discovered that the utilization of these procedures had increased, they reversed their course and decided to *lower* the reimbursement for outpatient procedures performed in doctors' offices and clinics not owned by the hospitals. The same hospitals began buying physicians' practices, along with their expensive, high-tech equipment, and installing the physicians' practices back into hospital-owned facilities where hospitals can charge more. On the one hand, it's a moral and societal problem: For elderly patients on fixed incomes, paying a double co-pay every time they see a specialist is an unsustainable increase, especially since elderly people often have chronic diseases that require ongoing monitoring and care. But the patients' complaints asking the physicians to move their offices out of the hospital and back across the street fall on deaf ears, due to the current financial incentives.

On the other hand, it's a financial dilemma for hospitals: How can they do anything but what they're doing? That's the problem with the legislative process when clinicians aren't involved. Regulations made with the best of intentions can lead to the worst of outcomes, and then new rules are instituted that lead to further unintended outcomes, requiring yet a new series of rules – and the vicious cycle of building more complexity and unworkability into the system continues.

It's terribly unfair to patients, but they can't simply go to a different hospital, because most hospitals are doing the same thing. Patients often can't find some other facility where they can avoid paying that extra co-pay for the facility fee. Many elderly patients can now afford their medications, but can't afford to see a doctor. For patients, it becomes a financial incentive not to see a doctor even when they need to, and perhaps to take medications when they don't.

The cost trap: a moving target

Our country has inherited a cost trap, after years of perpetuating the fee-for-service system. Consider pacemaker placement: In the early 1960s when pacemakers first became available, thoracic surgeons would implant them in the operating room. The pacemaker was relatively expensive, the size of a flattened softball, and the patient needed a day or two in the hospital to recover. The historical cost of that pacemaker has an effect on today's costs. Skip ahead to 2012; pacemakers are now the size of a quarter, and they're highly sophisticated computers. A cardiologist can implant them in a cardiac catheterization lab without an anesthesiologist, using only a local anesthetic, and the patient often goes home that same day. But the cost of implanting a pacemaker is now higher because the cardiologist's professional fees are based on historical physicians' fees. Complicating the problem, pacemaker companies now charge much more for their latest models to cover their research and development, further driving up overall costs.

The same thing happened with angioplasty. Initially, it was relatively well reimbursed, and insurance companies saw the benefit in paying cardiologists to perform angioplasties rather than a more expensive, complex surgery. But what was the real cost to a hospital to perform an angioplasty compared to surgery? When new technology comes in, the new procedure is compared to other procedures currently being done when assigned a payment amount in the DRG system. When doctors began to perform angioplasty, payments weren't analyzed in terms of what this or that component actually cost, but were instead assigned a payment relative to complex surgery.

Nontransparent actual costs

Health care has evolved as a nontransparent system, and no one wants to disclose the true costs. Historically, physicians charged what they wanted to be paid; later, the government and other insurers used those historical payments as a way to bundle payments to hospitals and fix the fee schedule for physicians.

But actual costs of care were never a factor in setting fees for physicians. When Medicare developed its Resource-Based Relative Value Scale to determine what it would reimburse physicians for various services, a key component was the "relative value unit," or RVU, an attempt to assign a certain value to a physician's work based on factors such as task complexity and physician time required. Other factors considered in Medicare reimbursement include practice expense and liability costs as well as geographic location.

But reimbursement formulas don't address or align with actual costs, which essentially remain invisible. Should costs ever be transparent? Perhaps consumers shouldn't care, just as they don't require that Toyota advertise the actual costs of its components to build each car. More than what a hospital's costs are to produce a given medical service, what really matters is what that service is worth: its value. If hospitals and doctors are paid a lump sum, even based on historical trends, and that payment is capped at a given level, healthcare inflation would start to disappear. Providers receiving that lump sum payment would have to evaluate their own processes and see how they can produce that service at a set cost.

Furthermore, suppose you did know the actual costs, what would you do with that data? Would you say to a physician, "We'll pay you cost plus 2%, 3%, or 5%? This has been the mentality of reform so far; these solutions are proposed extrinsically to the healthcare system. Wouldn't it be wiser for the federal government to decide what it's going to pay for overall health care and let providers figure out how to deliver that package in the most efficient way? The question of actual costs becomes irrelevant if you change the reimbursement scheme to create and pay for value.

DRGs (diagnosis-related groupings) succeeded in doing this for a while, until political will disappeared and Medicare began adding modifiers for procedures, essentially encouraging high-tech medicine again. Had Congress and Medicare had the discipline to say that they're not paying providers any more money, they would have forced providers to figure out, for instance, who really needs stents and how to place them cost-effectively. Instead, they agreed to putting in stents and paying more.

Because healthcare costs are not transparent, it's extremely difficult to gather accurate information about what a surgery or procedure actually costs a hospital or physician to perform. Going down the road of figuring out exactly what everything costs was part of the idea behind using "relative value units" to pay physicians. Medicare still employs this system of paying for more than 7,000 physician services based on a ranking of their "relative value" compared to other physician services, in terms of the physician's technical skill, time, judgment required, and stress to provide the service, as well as the practice expenses required behind the scenes, such as technology. The current system relies on CPT (current procedural terminology) codes to describe each physician service to calculate payment.

But trying to assess the actual costs for every kind of medical treatment doesn't address the problem of who would make the final decision about what the government would pay – or should pay, given clinical efficacy – for each service. My argument is that physicians, not bureaucrats, are in the best position to determine "relative value" clinically. Furthermore, increasing bureaucrats' control over physician behavior tends to trigger the natural reaction to rebel. Doctors have been successful because the process of going to medical school is essentially learning what the rules are and then learning how to win within the rules. If the rules change, the same sort of intelligence exists within people to look at the new rules and figure out how to win. All intelligent professionals do this; the stock market starts to crash, and intelligent investors see the new rules and change their tactics.

If you spend a lot of time analyzing costs, which various policy wonks do now, then what? Figuring out all of our healthcare system's actual costs and then deciding how to control costs would be an incredibly tedious process, fraught with all sorts of political fallout and scenarios that would be difficult to overcome. From a political perspective, it would never fly to say to the physicians who are now making $200,000 or $300,000 a year, "We've decided that you're now worth $60,000 because that's what doctors earn in other countries."

Projections based on historical costs

Only a modicum of solid ground for healthcare spending can be found in historical costs and cost-of-living increases. But that data is faulty; these analyses of "costs" are based on utilization patterns that were put into play historically and never based on actual costs, but instead based on the "usual and customary fees" that created free-for-all utilization patterns. We know that some of the historical trends are carrying "fat," so using historical data is shaky ground. In a sense we're already on unstable ground with evaluating healthcare costs, no matter who will decide the strategy of how to spend that money – government or a team of physicians.

Right now we're spending nearly 18% of GDP on health care, but the bigger issue is that it may be 25% of GDP in a few years – and we still don't know, as a country, what that number should be. It might be wiser to think of spending *x* percentage of GDP on health care to generate *y* dollars, and that's what we would pay for health care in this country per year. This model would cap spending. Over time, as the economy grows and healthcare spending stays flat or adjusts slightly for inflation, we'd have some control over costs. This kind of cost containment strategy could trickle down to hospital budgets as well. When a hospital decides how many MRI scanners it needs to buy, it's depreciating capital on a regular basis to plan for that; there's a cost involved. But if it knew that those projected costs were based on historical utilization patterns that ultimately needed to change, it could defer buying another scanner for a few years and save money. We've already tried tinkering with minor adjustments in physicians' fees, and it hasn't made a big enough difference. We have to take a longer view of health care and ask what could really work to control costs.

So what would work to control costs? A single-party payer could work; providers would gripe, but the beauty of a single-party payer is that it sets a budget, and that's the budget. The downside is having too many decisions made by a central committee instead of by the clinicians in the trenches doing the work. Instead, a better solution would be having a handful of integrated systems competing with each other in each state, for instance, rather than having Capitol Hill decide how much funding each state would receive with a state agency deciding how it will be distributed.

The cost of health care has grown 2% faster than the overall economy for the last 30 years, according to Ezekiel Emanuel, a former White House advisor and health policy expert, writing in *The New York Times* in October 2011. Ballooning costs end up being covered by borrowing money. The United States already spends $2.6 trillion a year on health care; continued growth at the current rate would make health care roughly one-third of the U.S. economy by 2035.

After researching and analyzing various reform ideas for cost containment, Emanuel and many other healthcare experts have concluded that one of the best solutions is to bundle payments to care for patients with multiple chronic diseases such as heart failure, emphysema, or diabetes. In fact, the least healthy 10% of patients spend 64% of our country's overall healthcare costs. But by integrating care – creating teams of physicians, nurses, care coordinators, and pharmacists to monitor patient care, including care in the home – providers have begun preventing these chronically ill patients from repeatedly bouncing back into the hospital. Preventing hospital and ED readmission carries with it significant cost savings. Bundling payments would cover a patient's entire "care episode" – a weeklong hospitalization or a two-day surgery stay – as a single payment, rather than paying for every CT scan, every x-ray, every doctor's bedside visit, every pill. The goal? Offer incentives for providers to work together, avoid duplication and unnecessary care, and provide safer care. Emanuel agrees with the need to end fee-for-service billing and its inherent incentives and move toward payers writing one check and letting providers figure it out.

The 1000-pound gorilla: physician utilization

Even after DRGs, hospital costs are still skyrocketing. Many healthcare economists and bureaucrats who design and implement DRGs argue that costs would have risen even higher without the diagnosis-related reimbursement scheme. Either way, it's clear that the DRG system hasn't controlled costs enough to keep the Medicare system solvent into the future. Hospitals can become more "efficient" with lots of nurses and managers running around with clipboards, figuring out how many days Aunt Jenny has stayed in the hospital, trying to get her out of the hospital and home as quickly as possible, making sure there's a cab for her, there's someone at home to help her, and she has all her medications.

All of that is valuable, but hospitals market it as "patient-centered care." This isn't really patient-centric care; it's DRG-centric care. Hospital leadership is under siege by the healthcare crisis as much as physicians are. *Pharmacy and Therapeutics*, a peer-reviewed journal for managed care and hospital drug formulary management, reported that the average hospital's supply costs alone rose almost 40% in just two years between 2003 and 2005. From a hospital CEO's perspective, the reality is that moving Aunt Jenny out of the hospital within the constraints of the DRG reimbursement system matters as much as what kind of care she receives. True patient-centric care, instead, would involve making decisions about the kinds of medical resources that Aunt Jenny needs along the continuum of care, and then providing them in the most cost-effective, collaborative way possible.

But the 1000-pound gorilla here, which hospitals still can't get under control, is physician utilization: the way doctors use all hospital-related resources. Once a patient is admitted to a hospital, his or her doctor essentially has complete discretion in what kind and how many of the hospital's services will be used, such as where the doctor admits the patient – a hugely expensive ICU bed, a less expensive regular bed in the hospital, or a still less expensive "observation" bed – and which diagnostic tests he or she orders, ranging from standard, hospital-admission lab tests to extensive use of MRI scans, nuclear imaging, and CT scans. Many of these costs are incurred before treatment even begins.

Physicians vary widely in how often they utilize expensive technology that has not been proven useful in patient care. There's tremendous variation in how often physicians order expensive diagnostic procedures and drugs when less-expensive tests or drugs might be just as – or more – effective. Physicians' use of hospital resources also varies widely in how often they admit patients to an expensive ICU setting when not needed, how quickly they transfer patients from high-cost centers of care to less expensive settings, and how quickly they make the right diagnosis and begin the right treatment. Tracking and controlling this kind of data on physician behavior poses a host of operational, clinical, and legal issues, given physicians' long-standing culture of autonomy, assumption of independence, and protection of their own and colleagues' turf when it comes to decision-making and patient care.

DRGs: failed hospital cost control

DRGs were originally designed to control hospital spending under Medicare Part A. When a patient is admitted to a hospital for the diagnostic code for congestive heart failure, for example, the hospital receives a fixed amount of money. Today, Medicare, Medicaid, and most private insurers prospectively pay the hospital for the "bundle" of services the hospital uses during a specific patient admission. The actual dollar amount for each DRG is subject to complex modifiers and adjustments over time. DRGs classify diseases by the patient's primary diagnosis, with the option to add up to eight secondary diagnoses and up to six procedures performed during a hospital stay.

For hospitals to receive payment under Medicare Part A, a physician documents the primary and secondary diagnoses and procedures; that data is then coded in the hospital's medical records department by a professional medical-record coder using the *International Classification of Diseases, Ninth Revision, Clinical Modification (ICD-9)*. The hospital submits that data to a fiscal intermediary, a company who contracts with Medicare to process and pay hospital claims under Medicare Part A. The fiscal intermediary inputs the data and runs it through an entirely different software system to review, sort, and process claims, called the Medicare Code Editor, which screens out cases that need further review prior to classifying them into one of the hundreds of different DRGs.

The system is further complicated by adding "relative weights" to each DRG, designed to account for the fact that some diagnoses require more hospital resources and are much more costly to treat than others. A case of life-threatening viral meningitis is more costly in hospital resources than a concussion, for instance, but much less costly than a heart transplant. The final DRG "relative weight" addresses cost-of-living adjustments, national cost averages, and multiple other factors.

Initially, hospital leadership grew anxious when DRGs began, knowing that hospitals traditionally have no control over physician utilization behavior and so couldn't put controls in place to make ends meet once Medicare capped its payments. Controlling the costs they could control proved to be an ineffective strategy for hospitals. Uncontrolled utilization and inefficiencies on the part of their independent physician staff, along with the rapid adoption of unproven and expensive technologies, continued to bend the hospitals' cost curve upward. So did the growth of outpatient facilities that could "cherry pick" patients with less-acute illnesses, forcing hospitals to take on primarily the sickest and most costly of patients.

Given their out-of-control costs, hospital leadership responded to the new Medicare DRGs by lobbying the government to give them more money, essentially trying to "un-cap" the capped payments of DRGs. And they succeeded. Now there are even more modifiers to the DRGs, so if a hospital admits a patient under the DRG for "congestive heart failure," and the patient also has another disease such as kidney failure, the hospital is paid more to admit that patient. For patients with a procedural code such as intracardiac stent placement, the hospital receives an even higher reimbursement.

Treating a patient with the DRG for acute ischemic stroke with thrombolysis, for example, used to cost hospitals more than they were reimbursed to provide that care. Now, with a new DRG to cover the procedure of thrombolysis, total payment for stroke increased from $5,000 to $11,500. The purpose of the DRG system – to help control healthcare spending – unraveled because hospitals had only limited control of their own costs. DRGs were never an effective strategy to control costs because the design was flawed to begin with. Hospitals couldn't survive on the original DRG prospective payment scheme, and they're barely surviving even now, after the adoption of more complicated payment modifiers; a hospital can't control costs generated by its physician staff, whose incentives are independent of, and at times in conflict with, the hospital.

Even today, the DRG system keeps growing more complicated. Now it's not just "congestive heart failure" – it's "congestive heart failure with renal insufficiency and cardiac catheterization," so there's the original two- or three-digit code plus everything that follows the decimal point, which modifies the reimbursement. That's why hospitals want physicians to be willing to document everything they do, so hospitals can add to the DRG coding – or "upcode" – to receive a higher reimbursement.

But most physicians lack a detailed awareness of the issues of billing for the hospital, or lack the time and motivation to fill out extra paperwork for the hospital's benefit. DRGs, which address only Medicare Part A, may continue to stimulate the economy for Medicare coders and bureaucrats, but they can't control overall Medicare costs that are, by definition, beyond the control of the Part A beneficiaries – the hospitals.

Here's the other fly in the ointment: Every time the government adds another level of detail and administration to the system, it creates yet another layer of bureaucracy that costs the country money. Every hospital now has to hire professional "medical coders" who are trained to read through a patient's medical chart during a hospital admission; it's a fairly sophisticated task, they're paid a professional-level salary, and hospitals can't afford to hire a lot of them.

Their work is made more difficult because most hospitals still use paper charts. In one survey published in *The New England Journal of Medicine* in 2009, only 1.5% of hospitals in the United States had electronic medical records systems in all clinical units. In most current hospital systems, medical coders look through each page of a paper-based patient chart, making sure that everything billable is billed for and documented; and nothing's being billed for that hasn't been documented. There aren't enough trained medical coders; many become burned out and move on to other careers, and hospitals are left rehiring, retraining – or outsourcing the work to India. It's a stressful, tedious job, as well as technical, because if a hospital bills for care that's not documented, that's considered "Medicare fraud and abuse." Hospitals bear the financial risk of their DRG billing, while physicians only bear the risk for being falsely charged with "fraud and abuse" with their own billings, since Medicare pays them separately in the fee-for-service system under Medicare Part B.

Employing physicians: an incomplete fix

DRGs didn't fix the utilization or cost problem, so hospital leadership began looking for the next big idea and decided to start employing their physicians, thinking that would solve the cost problem. But it doesn't for two reasons. First, "perverse incentives" still make it in a hospital's best interests for its physicians to provide more care so they can bill more. When hospitals employ physicians, outside of a few self-insured systems such as Group Health in Seattle and Kaiser-Permanente in California, the hospitals essentially become collecting agencies for the physicians' professional fees.

Second, employing physicians doesn't control costs because doctors can easily maneuver around regulations, if they choose to, so the regulatory environment has misfired here as well. Most states have clauses in their hospitals' contracts that limit the hospital from interfering with a physician's medical judgment about what's best for his or her patient. A physician whose utilization pattern is far more costly than his average peer can successfully argue that his pattern was due to his best medical judgment. The bottom line: It's almost impossible for a hospital to control a doctor's utilization behavior in its facility – or the economic impact of that behavior – because of the liability issue. The doctor could retaliate by saying, "They're not allowing me to practice medicine and do what's best for my patients." It's a tough argument for hospitals to win.

So while the majority of physicians are now employed, it's not going to solve the overall cost problem, because the physician reimbursement system is still based on fee-for-service. There's an intense economic conflict at play: The less a hospital spends to treat a patient, the more money the hospital makes. The more care and services the doctor provides, the more income he or she earns.

Cost-shifting in hospitals

A critical symptom of the fiscal crisis in health care is the rise of cost-shifting in health care over the past several years. Because Medicaid and Medicare typically don't pay enough for hospitals to make a profit, hospitals tend to shift costs onto private payers or uninsured people. Uninsured patients might see hospital bills where an IV is billed at

$3,000; since they're paying out-of-pocket, they're paying "retail" costs, whereas if they had insurance, they'd pay "wholesale." The healthcare provider has negotiated a discounted rate with Medicare and all the insurance companies who are competing with each other by offering lower costs.

There's a shell game going on in hospitals as they try to balance their budgets, but cost-shifting makes it nearly impossible to solve the overall cost problem, since actual costs of medical services have become so varied – and remain hidden. Healthcare pricing is similar to the sticker price on a new car: Some individual consumers may get discounts, fleet purchases extract significant discounts, and no one seems to know how the total price was determined or what "undercoating" and other extra services mean. But while there are sources such as Consumer Reports that allow the purchaser to see the dealer's actual cost, similar comparative cost data is almost impossible to obtain in health care.

As an illustrative anecdote, when my son recently became ill in California and was severely dehydrated and needed some IV fluids, he went to a free-standing emergency clinic, was given a liter of IV saline, and sent home. I received a bill for $10,000, with $3,000 worth of IVs. How much does salt water actually cost? That same $10,000 bill, when submitted to an insurer, would have been processed at a prediscounted rate of perhaps $2,000; and after review, the private insurer might decide it was only worth $1,800, and only pay $1,800 – and the hospital would have taken the check.

Hospitals and insurers negotiate rates before the contract is signed, and discounts are then fixed for the duration of the contract. Most states have tried unsuccessfully to regulate how much hospitals can charge individuals, but because of the intense economic pressure on hospitals from their discounted revenues, current regulations certainly aren't adequate in keeping hospitals from using "retail" pricing whenever possible, which hits hard on people who don't have insurance. That's one of the reasons why, when people go into debt for health care, it's so overwhelming. An individual can owe a hospital and its physicians tens or even hundreds of thousands of dollars after a catastrophic medical illness, wiping out any family savings and sending them into bankruptcy.

The rising costs of healthcare policing

"Eliminating Medicare fraud and abuse" plays a key role in some politicians' strategies as a proposed way to save money. The fear of fraud and abuse horrifies hospital leadership; the last thing they want is to see a federal agency descend upon them, open up their records forever, essentially hamstringing them for several days while they're trying to find more "fraud and abuse." Not to mention what happens if the local news reports that one of its major hospitals is being investigated for fraud and abuse. The hospital's public relations and reputation are hit hard, especially if the inquiry is also reported in the national websites that rank hospitals.

The government makes the hospitals' coding, reporting, and billing systems more complicated every year, so there are more cases of mistaken fraud and abuse every year. While the front end of the "policing" system includes hospitals now paying for medical coders to check coding and billing, the back end of the system is patrolled by federal employees looking for fraud and abuse through programs created in 1996. To enhance these "program integrity" efforts for Medicare, Congress approved additional discretionary funding of $198 million for fiscal year 2009 and $311 million for fiscal year 2010.

More policing won't lower national healthcare costs; it will increase costs by adding layers of administrators. Even more frustrating for Americans footing the bill: None of that money touches a patient, improves patient care, or funds high-value technology. The Affordable Care Act signed into law in 2010 will likely make this problem worse, by increasing the need to pay a sizable staff of medical coders and federal agents for oversight. From its inception in 1997, the federal Health Care Fraud and Abuse Control (HCFAC) program has invested in investigations, enforcement, and audits run through the Office of the Inspector General, Department of Justice, and FBI. New HCFAC funding – $10 million a year for 10 years in fiscal years 2011 through 2020, and an additional $250 million spread across fiscal years 2011 to 2016 through the Health Care and Education Reconciliation Act of 2010 – is targeted to expand Medicare and Medicaid investigations, audits, and compliance.

The balkanization of medicine

Because of the absence of a value proposition in health care today, the competition among all sectors is based on gaming the financial incentive system currently in place. We've created an untenable balkanization of medicine, with multiple, competing interests fighting to take their share of a limited pie, without a shared sense of the big picture and mindset that asks: Is there enough pie to go around?

The balkanization of medicine has made the American Medical Association nearly obsolete; less than one-third of physicians in the United States now belong to the AMA. The effective physician lobbies have become the specialty lobbies: the American Academy of Family Physicians, American College of Cardiology, American College of Ophthalmology, American College of Radiology, American Urological Association, and others. Every specialty hires professional political lobbyists as well as pays physicians to lobby constantly on Capitol Hill. Even university physicians have their own lobby. Physicians are competing among themselves to avoid more reimbursement cuts to their specialty, so every specialty's message to Congress is the same: "Don't cut us."

Physician specialty groups are not alone in their proprietary lobbying efforts. The insurance industry, pharmaceutical industry, device makers, nurses, and other special interests are all in D.C., fighting for themselves. These lobbyists, all claiming to represent the best interests of the patient, try to persuade Congress to maintain the maximum reimbursement for their part of the healthcare budget – typically without addressing the overall issues in healthcare spending today.

In their presentations, they argue for "better patient care," and their rationale is that cutting their reimbursement means they can't take care of patients. They argue, "If you cut my reimbursement, I can't see

Medicare patients," or "I can't spend the kind of time I need to spend with Medicare patients, since I need to see more of them to make ends meet and make up for the shortfall." That's not disingenuous; it's true. But when I've sat down to talk with them, they don't seem to see this as a shortsighted way of looking out for themselves.

Their arguments don't address the big picture; the specialty lobbyists aren't asking Congress to focus on the urgent national issue of how to control costs and create value. Their primary focus is to assure that their own reimbursement isn't cut. They're not spending time suggesting where else they might cut costs in how they provide care, and they're not getting paid to propose better overall solutions to healthcare reform.

Healthcare systems, as well, are competing among themselves for patients instead of looking at the overall population of an area and strategically evaluating how to take care of that population in a high-quality, cost-effective way. This competition isn't driving down costs; it's increasing costs. One hospital wants to take the highest-paying patients away from another, so it builds an expensive, high-tech, free-standing Emergency Department when there's already a new, high-tech ED in that same town. Now that town has two expensive facilities, both reimbursed by Medicare and private insurers at good rates, and both spending time, money, and intellectual resources going after the same limited pool of patients in that community.

Competition in medicine also shows up in the shortage of medical schools in this country, which is projected to become increasingly worse and contribute to the national shortage of practicing physicians. It's difficult to build new medical schools due to the significant expense and the resistance of established medical schools. The dean of one medical school could argue that it would dilute the quality of medical education if another medical school is built nearby and wouldn't be in the best interests of patients for the state to license another medical school. In reality, fewer medical schools creates a higher demand for new physicians and their services, allowing doctors – practically requiring them – to be well paid to pay off their medical school debt, further exacerbating the national crisis in healthcare spending.

A pundit once quipped that attacking health care is like punching jello; it just bulges out somewhere else. So the specialty lobbies continue to compete with their colleagues without an overall, integrated strategy that will lead our country into the future and be sustainable in the long run.

Medicare entitlement, Medicare bankruptcy

Because Medicare is an entitlement, it's an extremely difficult system to change. Once the public has an expectation that society owes them something or they have earned it, and once beneficiaries of federal entitlement funding become numerous and politically active, as with Medicare, anyone trying to change that entitlement will meet with tremendous resistance. In fact, Medicare played a major role in allowing the entitlement concept to take root, along with other social programs such as social security. Historically, when Americans paid little in the way of income tax, they had little in the way of expectations from the government. As government grew and played a larger role in Americans' daily lives, the sense of entitlement – and dependency on the government – increased.

Lyndon Johnson started several programs that became entitlements – federal money for education, school lunches, and federal welfare and disability insurance programs – expanding the role of government rapidly in the 1960s. Medicare, part of a series of programs that have contributed to the entitlement mentality, has grown into a wild beast due to its size – and political clout. Cut school lunches for kids from the federal budget and you'd save a tiny percentage of the overall budget; but cut Medicare and you'd cut a huge percentage. In 2010, the three major health insurance programs – Medicare, Medicaid, and the Children's Health Insurance Program (CHIP) – together accounted for 21% of the budget, or $732 billion. Almost two-thirds of that, or $452 billion, went to Medicare, which accounted for fully 14% of the 2011 federal budget.

Economists can't decide when Medicare will go bankrupt because there's been a shell game going on all along for Medicare funding, shuffling money back and forth among funds and borrowing from the Medicare trust fund to keep itself afloat. It has become impossible to pinpoint with certainty when Medicare will go belly-up. The Congressional Budget Office (CBO) and Centers for Medicare and Medicaid (CMS) have frequently revised their estimates about future costs, so clearly it's a moving target. Just how much of a moving target it is, given the complexity of the system, may still be unknown. According to CMS, Medicare enrollees *doubled* to 47 million between 1975 and 2010, while the real cost to cover them *quadrupled*. Further, CMS estimates that Medicare will nearly double again by 2040 to cover 88 million enrollees – and at a cost three times higher than in 2010.

The reality, then, is that politicians and policy makers working on healthcare reform have to figure out not only how to continue providing adequate medical care to seniors, but also how to control Medicare's spiraling costs and make it financially sustainable in the long run. But many politicians aren't willing to say that Medicare is the problem; it's a political nightmare. In 2011, when Paul Ryan (R-WI), Chairman of the Congressional House Budget Committee, declared that healthcare reform won't work without making some changes to entitlements, specifically Medicare, the Democrats came out firing with media sound bites targeted to seniors, claiming that the Republicans were going to destroy Medicare. Republicans and Democrats alike have been similarly attacked verbally by senior voters, yelling that politicians were taking Medicare away, when in fact most proposals being considered wouldn't touch entitlements to current seniors. When it comes to the healthcare debate in the media, facts often don't lead the story. It's become such a volatile issue, with both parties trying to benefit and push their agendas by polarizing and misreporting the facts.

Sound bite: denying claims

In promoting the healthcare reform legislation of 2010, politicians claimed that they would go after insurance companies who spend more money denying claims than paying them. That's another sound bite distortion of reality, but it plays well with consumers, since most Americans have had trouble at some time trying to get an insurer to pay for a medical procedure. Denying coverage, for consumers, usually happens because a procedure wasn't coded correctly or the details of insurance benefits, outlined in their policies, weren't followed.

From the insurers' perspective, they're selling an insurance product for a set amount based on what that product covers. If their product doesn't cover bone marrow transplantation and says so in their published outline of benefits, for a patient to buy that product and then say they're being "denied coverage" for bone marrow transplant isn't really fair. You can't buy a car without an air conditioner and then try to make a legal complaint that the air conditioner doesn't work.

For a politician to say that insurance companies are spending more money denying claims than paying them is a distortion of the issue. In 2008, for example, total national health expenditures in the United States exceeded $2.3 trillion. Of that, $92 billion went for the cost, overhead, and profit of private health insurance. Even assuming that insurance companies' overhead and profits were all focused on "denying claims," their administrative cost accounted for only 3.9% of the 2008 budget. Professional services – doctors, nurses, dentists, and other clinical services – accounted for 31.3% of the $2.3 trillion, hospitals accounted for 30.7%, and retail sales of drugs and other medical products accounted for 12.8%.

Large, national media organizations using focus groups know precisely what will resonate with consumers and how to create effective sound bites, however misleading, to shape public opinion. If a sound bite claims that insurers spend more money denying than paying claims, public opinion can be easily swayed unless consumers educate themselves on healthcare issues.

The failure of politics as primary change agent

The way the political process works, members of Congress are focused on piecemeal solutions. They want to repeal the sustainable growth rate formula for physician payment so they don't alienate their physician constituents, but its repeal would result in an increase in Medicare spending that further jeopardizes its sustainability. Instead, there's a more far-sighted kind of physician leadership possible among physician colleagues. It's now time to step back and ask how we can actually fix our healthcare system, not with a bandaid here or minor legislation there, but with a systemic change that will work long-term to stop the financial hemorrhaging. Our country has backed itself into a corner where the only options to resolve the healthcare crisis for good are all painful – and they're especially painful for politicians. For a member of Congress to come out and tell the truth about healthcare spending and the current Medicare crisis, he or she would have to accept that they're not likely to be reelected.

The Clinton administration took the first step in starting the national dialog about the healthcare crisis. From a physician's perspective, there were plenty of problems with the plan Clinton proposed, but it was worth discussing. Unfortunately, the "Harry and Louise" political ads from the Health Insurance Association of America killed the discussion, scaring people that bureaucrats and not doctors would be making key decisions about their health care. It's a great example of a sound bite winning against a rational debate of the complex issues. Some strategists might say that it was political suicide for Bill Clinton to stand up and declare that it was time to talk about health care; but at least he initiated and furthered the conversation that began to educate the American public at large.

The needed conversation still isn't happening. Even the current national dialog fails to focus enough on health care in terms of its *value* and *affordability*; recent reforms primarily focus on *access*. But the bigger problem is not access; it's not the uninsured; it's *cost* and *value*. Having so many Americans uninsured is an ethical and societal problem, but that's not the operational misfiring at the heart of the healthcare system. Resolving the healthcare crisis requires the creation of value in health care, which will require a transformative change in how much we pay, and how we pay, for medical services. The value issue remains a daunting prospect that few politicians want to take on and face squarely and openly.

The reality is that to fix Medicare, especially as a president or presidential candidate, means making a lot of people extremely unhappy. It's still the right thing to do, but no president would be reelected after coming out and saying that we as a country cannot afford to spend nearly 18% of our GDP on health care, and that we need to bring it down to 10% or 12% – or at the very least, not allow it to grow to a larger percentage – to be competitive in the global market. Further, that president would have to commit considerable resources to the problem, mobilize every healthcare agency involved, and focus a huge majority of government staff, time, effort, and discussion around the healthcare crisis.

If a president ever took that strong of a stand for health care, the next day you'd see vehemently negative political ads and a host of outrageous Internet videos. Specialty physician lobbies would pour huge funds into campaigns to preserve their independence and fees. The unions would likely refuse to see health care as anything but a hard-won entitlement. Insurance companies would protect their interests in the status quo along with pharmaceutical and medical device companies. The AARP would lobby hard to preserve its entitlement.

Health care came up on the national radar screen in an entirely new way with President Clinton, which was courageous of him since he must have known he was going to be politically mauled. Thanks to him, more Americans are aware of the complexity and entanglements in the rat's nest of health care. Unfortunately, the failure of the Clinton initiative remains embedded in every politician's mind. Democrat or Republican, they don't want to be shredded like Clinton was, and you can't blame them. In the absence of physicians moving reform forward in a more rational way, our country will likely end up with a mirror of the Canadian healthcare system. True, Americans don't like waiting in line, but, in the absence of physician leadership focused on creating value, our political process will guarantee that we'll soon be in such a fiscal crisis that a single-party-payer system may be the only option.

The health care crisis isn't likely to be answered politically; it's a no-win situation for politicians. Reform has to come from strong physician leadership backed by functional financial and political incentives so doctors can begin to engage more actively with the future of health care, create value in health care, and design sane ways of reaching those goals.

CHAPTER 3
Reframing the Debate

Health care as a national concern is comparable to the energy debate: a hugely complicated issue that's not being shaped in a viable way. "Sustainable energy," for instance, sounds great as an idea, but we can't continue to drive the way we drive, commute the way we commute, and sustain those current lifestyles only on solar and wind power. The environmental movement has seized on the idea of sustainable energy, and everything else is a no-go; while the oil lobby has seized on the idea that our country has plenty of oil and just needs to drill for it. Thus the energy issue isn't being shaped the way the problem ought to be shaped: Oil is a strategic commodity that's killing our country.

A similar dynamic is happening in health care: No one's shaping the problem realistically. The fact is that American medicine is a strategic commodity that's killing us. We can't continue to incentivize doctors to overutilize healthcare resources, add DRG modifiers that increase and further complicate Medicare payments, increase baby boomer enrollees in Medicare, increase access to care for the currently uninsured by adding millions of new Medicaid enrollees, adopt and reimburse unproven expensive new technologies and medications, burden businesses with skyrocketing healthcare premiums, raise consumers' premiums and co-pays every year – and still sustain our country's economy. The current crisis in health care can only be resolved in the long run by reframing the issues in ways that keep both clinical and financial realities in mind.

Physicians produce value, regulations produce bureaucrats

One could argue that if a medical service or product is worth *x*, and we expect certain standards from that service, then what role should government or insurers play in how it's produced? Should they care how physicians or hospitals do their business internally? If hospitals choose to have physicians on contract, or put them on salaries, or pay them for certain things and not for others, why should government or consumers care, as long as physicians are producing a valued service at agreed-upon standards of care?

It's counterproductive to waste the expensive time of practicing physicians in navigating the myriad of regulatory burdens imposed on them by government agencies and insurers, all trying to tell the medical profession how to produce their "product" – health care – without a clear vision of what the country actually wants, needs, and values. That's the fundamental problem many physicians and hospital leaders have with the Affordable Care Act of 2010: It's overfilled with micromanagement, without an overall, new vision of health care.

Instead, we as a society need to step back and agree on what we need for health care as a society and what we're willing to pay for it, as a country and as individuals. Will we let healthcare spending rise to 25% or 30% of GDP, or put the brakes on spending? Whatever form the solution may take, we should let physician leaders who understand patient care work together and figure out how to deliver that care at that cost.

That's how you develop great products, not by micromanaging people. Few people would argue with the results Steve Jobs achieved; successful innovators such as Apple hire smart executives who don't tell people how to produce their products. Instead, they've inspired people around the world to work in garages producing "apps" and other Apple products, and Apple ends up wildly successful as the middleman with the platform. The same creative thinking and leadership can propel the healthcare industry into new forms of innovation and success.

Defining value: quality divided by cost

How do we define value in health care? What we've come to expect and accept is driven largely by the culture, history, and traditions of U.S. health care, which has become convenience-oriented and market-share oriented – two qualities that, by definition, encourage unnecessary costs. "What we want" tends to be what we've grown used to, while "what we need" would instead focus on a baseline of medical services that assures the overall health of the country.

Value is generally defined as quality divided by cost. When we evaluate healthcare reform proposals as a nation, of course we want quality, but we don't have unlimited funds. Since our national budget for health care must have limits, how do we produce more value? One mindset looks at what you're producing and makes sure that you're not spending any money on factors that don't add to quality. But this approach could lead to adding more layers of bureaucrats as an oversight function. The more proactive, positive approach would be to evaluate what you're producing and make sure that you *are* spending money on factors that add to quality – the intelligent role for physicians on the ground.

Currently, with the fee-for-service reimbursement structure, there's little incentive to do that analysis. But we have the successful model of DRGs (diagnostic-related groupings) in hospitals: As soon as Medicare fixed hospital reimbursements in a "bundled service" model, hospital staff concentrated a lot more on value. Redundant, unnecessary hospitals went out of business, others scaled back considerably, and still others morphed into different facilities such as nursing homes. Hospital operations underwent consolidation and a marked change in staffing ratios; nurses expressed concern about reduced quality of care in lowering the nurse-to-patient ratios, but objective outcomes data doesn't support that.

What this points out is the difference between the "hard" data of morbidity and mortality versus "soft" data on quality of care, including convenience and patient satisfaction. Which data are we as a society going to use, moving forward with reform? The fact is that morbidity and mortality rates in our country keep dropping; they didn't rise, for instance, with a change in nurse-to-patient ratios. True, it's more stressful for the nurses and for patients. Some families who can afford it now hire a private nurse for a family member in the hospital. Private nurses offer a value proposition, since families recognize that what's being offered in some hospitals makes it worthwhile to pay for a private nurse.

When DRGs forced hospitals to reduce their costs, they began looking at utilization of their own resources, particularly the length of hospital stays. They began evaluating what a length of stay should look like for each medical problem and how to reduce length of stay, the biggest factor in hospital costs.

Cardiologists now implant pacemakers with only an overnight stay, while we used to keep patients in the hospital for two or three days. Patients after heart attacks now go home in several days; they used to spend two weeks in the hospital. There's no data to suggest that a shorter hospital stay means a lower quality of care; in fact, in some cases a shorter hospitalization means better care. When the system pushed cardiovascular surgeons to get patients moving sooner after surgery, the patients were actually healthier, because by extubating (removing the endotracheal tube) patients earlier, patients did better and had fewer postoperative complications. By getting patients up and around more quickly after many surgeries, such as hip or knee replacement surgery, their risk of infection and lung clots decreased. Those positive outcomes led to moving patients through other hospitalizations more quickly, as well.

So while it's difficult as a society to define value in health care, the reality is that we can no longer avoid it and resolve the fiscal healthcare crisis. Setting limits on what we're spending and letting physicians lead the way in figuring out how to best spend those funds would be a good start. After listening to the reactions and perspectives of patients to keep the process balanced, we'd end up with more value for our healthcare dollars than we have now.

Part of the value equation also means defining quality – another essential role for physician leaders. There are so many different perspectives of what "quality" means – perspectives from the patient, the doctor, the hospital, the insurer – but if you start cutting costs without negatively affecting objective outcomes such as morbidity and mortality, it's hard to argue that you've cut quality. In the case of shorter hospital stays, as noted, cutting costs seems to improve quality. Using protocols for antibiotic selection reduced the number of drug-resistant organisms and lowered overall drug cost, since often the most effective antibiotic is also the least expensive.

When you consider overall utilization of healthcare resources, getting people out of the hospital and home as soon as it's safe to discharge them is a good example of how to improve quality and reduce cost. From a patient's perspective, hospitals aren't the best places to recuperate; and most people, unless they live alone or have no social support, would much rather be at home. So if you get people through complicated procedures quicker, and home faster, and back to work sooner – those are factors in defining "quality." You've certainly cut a lot of waste and therefore cost. Hospital discharge is clearly a patient-by-patient determination as far as readiness to go home, but it's hard to argue with a measure that improves patient outcomes while cutting waste.

Physicians, nurses, and most healthcare leaders I've met aren't going to jeopardize patient care. It's simply not part of the medical culture; it's just not in their nature. The medical community would rebel before purposely cutting corners and accepting worse patient outcomes. Hospitals proved this during the advent of DRGs, when Medicare limited their funds and hospital leaders had to find ways to cut fat out of their costs without cutting muscle. At times, muscle was cut, and hospital and physician leaders quickly revisited their operations to restore the muscle of patient care.

Defining quality and value includes pushing clinicians to evaluate everything they do related to patient care, what's needed and not needed, every time they touch a patient. It would be a long process, but we'd end up with a better healthcare system than if we let the government and political system dictate the future healthcare system without putting the national budget at the forefront of the debate. Consider what the government has done with healthcare spending over the last 20 years: Chiropractic, acupuncture, massage therapy, and wheelchairs are all included. TV ads for motorized scooters tell consumers that if they're on Medicare, they can have one for free; the advertiser will figure out how to bill their insurance so patients don't have to pay for anything. To physicians, that's off-target and hugely wasteful. If a patient can't walk with a cane or walker and can't navigate in a wheelchair, then he or she needs a motor scooter – but not everyone on Medicare needs one. The system can't afford to pay for everyone to have one; some patients may have to spend their own money and buy their own motor scooter if they want convenience that's not medically necessary.

The point is that no one understands medical necessity better than physicians: not the insurers, not the pharmaceutical companies, and not the device companies, who all have strong financial incentives to push patients toward a certain treatment that favors their own bottom lines. Physicians have a much better idea of who needs a given treatment or medical device than administrators at Medicare.

Overproduction in health care

Understanding overproduction is central to the need to reframe the healthcare debate. The problem lies in too often allowing the healthcare debate to revolve around the individual's use of health care, such as politicians' sound bites of one patient's medical horror story or how many MRIs are performed on how many individual people. But a much larger factor in the equation here is that we're manufacturing redundant medical technology that's unnecessary, costly, and isn't making a real contribution to our nation's overall health, from new MRI scanners to capital-intensive, free-standing EDs.

By way of contrast, healthcare providers in each province in Canada receive a set amount of money to provide care each year, and they have to decide how many of a given procedure or diagnostic test, such as an MRI, they need to do while still staying within those limits. Canada performs far fewer MRIs than in the United States due to the differing reimbursement systems. American physicians can bill for every scan they do and get paid for it, so the clear temptation is to buy more scanners and do more scans.

This illustrates how health care is not a free market. If a car manufacturer produces too many cars, they sit on the lot, and eventually the dealer has to cut prices to move them. If the auto industry was designed as health care is now, car manufacturers would be paid a fixed price for every car they produced, regardless of whether it was needed or not, and they'd just go on producing cars. If there's no financial incentive not to overproduce, industries tend to overproduce.

Because policy makers are locked into a fee-for-service mentality that underlies most healthcare reform, all of their assumptions are based on previous, often dubious data – which makes healthcare planning a house of cards. If the number of MRI machines grew one year by 15%, they predict what that percentage of growth will be in the future – rather than stopping to reevaluate the use of MRI and realize that the system may not need another one for a long time. Analysts look at it like you'd look at a typical market: You have historical data and try to project based on demographics and other key data points. Without challenging the underlying assumptions, those projections are illusory.

By analyzing reports from the White House Office of Management and Budget (OMB) that try to project long-term Medicare, Medicaid, and total healthcare spending, it's clear just how much analysts don't know. Those OMB reports and projections are typically built on a host of "what ifs" and assumptions that aren't grounded in how clinical medicine is actually practiced. The OMB ends up spending time analyzing data based on an entirely incomplete way of thinking, using historical trends and costs. The real question is: Given a fixed amount of money, how can we as a society get the biggest bang for the buck in terms of the country's overall health? That's what value is all about. Consumers as well as policy makers need to look at the assumptions our healthcare spending is built around to see the house of cards we've built.

Coronary stenting: a case of overproduction

How did it happen that our country spends an enormous amount of money on elective coronary stenting when studies suggest that it has no benefit in terms of preventing heart attack or promoting longevity? It's because of the financial incentives associated with doing stent procedures. When a new medical technology arrives on the scene, hospitals and providers get excited about it – and it's especially exciting when they can make money on it. Device labs make money manufacturing the stents, sales reps make money selling them, cardiologists make money doing the procedures to put the stents in, and hospitals and multispecialty clinics make money providing the facility in which to do the procedures. The new technology generates jobs that pay decent salaries.

Then the data comes out showing that stents don't prevent heart attacks or improve longevity. Instead of putting a moratorium on the new technology to reevaluate whether it's the right way to go, there are more stent procedures performed the following year, not fewer. The device company comes out with a new stent it claims addresses the issues with the previous version, such as a new "non-occluding" stent that won't eventually lead to new blockage in the artery.

The reality is that we now know that the underlying disease process isn't simply a function of blockage. It's not intuitively obvious, but the data suggests that the real mechanism of heart attack and sudden death is not necessarily the degree of narrowing in the artery per se, as physicians have thought for many years, but the amount of plaque throughout the artery – the plaque "burden." But medical procedures and payments have been built around that assumption of narrowing, so it's going to be difficult to change. The question becomes how to fold new clinical research into clinical practice more consistently and effectively – again, a good argument for physician leaders. With medical devices, the FDA looks at safety, not efficacy or value. Physician leadership could play a central role in restructuring the clinical trials process, perhaps in the direction of conducting clinical trials before new technology is approved to evaluate value as well as safety.

New medical knowledge shows that the real mechanism of heart attack lies in the endothelium (the lining of the blood vessel), which turns out to be an active, key player in the process; it does more than simply allow the transmission of blood back and forth. Any injury within the vessel starts the atherosclerotic process, but it's the inflammatory reaction to the injury by the endothelial cells that actually causes blood clot formation, blockage in the artery, and heart attack. A 40% to 50% obstruction in an artery is essentially undetectable by noninvasive cardiac imaging such as a nuclear stress test or stress echocardiogram; so no matter how much money you spend on diagnostic testing, those tests won't detect that stenosis. You might find it with a CT scan, but because CT scanning was never well reimbursed, it isn't typically used.

But with a 40% stenosis, if you have a fight with your spouse, your levels of the stress hormone epinephrine can rise and the atherosclerotic plaque can rupture, which attracts the blood platelets and forms the clots that cause the sudden closure in the artery of a heart attack. Stents treat only a small segment of the artery and actually cause inflammation when placed in the vessel. While this acute inflammation can be mitigated by embedding anti-inflammatory agents in the stent itself – the so-called drug-eluding stents – the overall atherosclerotic process in the rest of the vessel is unaffected by stent placement. It's not surprising, therefore, to see the data showing that stenting doesn't prevent heart attacks or prolong life.

To prevent heart attacks, if you look at what really makes a difference – such as the new statins, the drugs that lower cholesterol – they seem to work as anti-inflammatory and membrane-stabilizing agents as well as cholesterol-lowering agents. No one knows for sure which of these statin effects is most important, but when people with heart disease who have normal cholesterol levels are put on statins, they consistently have better outcomes. Some physicians have even gone so far as to suggest that the country might be better off putting every male who turns 50 on a statin and an aspirin, and not doing all the diagnostic testing we're currently doing. While this proposal hasn't been tested, it's the kind of value-driven thinking that leads to sound management of the national budget and maximizing value from healthcare dollars.

As a cardiologist, I've watched as new technology is introduced over the years and seen the difference between how it's adopted into private-practice offices versus hospitals. While high-tech specialties affiliated with a hospital are working with the latest diagnostic imaging or other technology, some primary care doctors in private practice have to work with an old Rube Goldberg contraption due to the financial realities of reimbursement. Physicians in the hospital tend to take the position that they don't want to be involved in making decisions involving finance; they don't see that as their job. In fact, physicians in private practice do that all the time; most run a lean office. To avoid compromising quality of care and to provide more consistent care across populations, physician leaders across multiple specialties should be involved in the analysis of the most effective use of technology.

The CT story: a study in underproduction

Based on current financial incentives, our healthcare system not only overutilizes some technologies but also underutilizes others. The recent history of CT scanning clearly illustrates how the healthcare industry works in this country, how potentially worthwhile technologies can be underproduced in a climate that rewards other, more expensive technology. The old calcium CT scanners (EBT, or "Ultrafast CT scanning") arrived on the scene in 1983, just before coronary stenting started in 1986. An algorithm was developed for using the new CT to diagnose atherosclerosis. A patient would hold his or her breath while

CT images of the heart were taken that could detect minute amounts of calcium in the coronary arteries.

From a practical standpoint in the United States, if you have calcium in your coronary arteries, you have coronary disease. The calcium isn't a "risk factor," you're not "at risk" for atherosclerosis; you already have coronary disease. I participated in a calcium-scanning study with B. Greg Brown, MD, and the University of Washington that began in the mid-1990s and was published in 2001. The research showed that calcium scans were more predictive of coronary severity than traditional risk-factor analysis.

But during that same time, the technology for stenting was released, along with the technology for intracoronary ultrasound, which allows cardiologists to put minute catheters into the arteries to image the inside of a blood vessel. The intracoronary ultrasound technology is "sexier" than looking at calcium scans – for the providers, the media, and consumers. The insurance companies, of course, didn't want to pay for either the new calcium scanning or the stenting technologies. But while EBT was developed by a small company with little or no influence, stents and intracoronary ultrasound were developed by large companies with political clout. Stents were reimbursed, and their utilization skyrocketed.

CT scanning, on the other hand, never really took off, and to this day clinical researchers haven't fully explored the potential of using CT scanning to diagnose heart disease, figure out whom to treat and not treat, or improve patients' longevity and quality of care. The hard reality here is that decisions about new technology adoption are often more influenced by well-financed industry lobbying than on an objective value paradigm.

Conflicts of interest: self-referrals

Specialty care has clearly contributed to major advances in U.S. health care over the past several decades. Hundreds of thousands of lives have been saved or significantly enhanced by endoscopic discovery of precancerous lesions, permanent pacemaker implantation, kidney transplantation, bone marrow transplantation, joint replacement, laser-based retinal surgery, neonatal intensive care units, and other advances in specialty care. But when technologies and specialties are closely linked by profitability-per-procedure, health care can become less about the patients' interests and more about the scramble for dollars. Too many doctors still don't fully appreciate the conflict of interest between how they want to practice medicine autonomously and how that impacts the entire healthcare system.

In the past, physicians had far fewer conflicts of interest. You went to your family doctor for your medical needs, and your family doctor would decide if you needed further care. If you needed surgery, he or she would refer you to a surgeon, so there was a built-in "second opinion" by the family doctor, which essentially protected patients from unnecessary surgeries. You knew when you walked into the surgeon's office that you'd already been evaluated by your primary care physician, who had no economic interest in the surgery itself.

Compare that to what happens in a typical cardiologist's office today. A patient walks in with chest pain, the cardiologist evaluates the patient, and then refers the patient back to his or her own practice for a diagnostic test or invasive intervention that the cardiologist makes money on. That's a built-in conflict of interest. Practicing cardiologists might argue that it's better for the patient because it's "one-stop shopping," more efficient and convenient for patients. While there may be some truth to that for a few patients, it defies logic to suggest that there isn't a conflict of interest that can create problems.

In fact, the literature is filled with reports of egregious use of self-referral. The cardiologist in the Baltimore-area hospital mentioned earlier who dramatically overutilized stents illustrates an outrageous case of providing unnecessary care – one that doctor profited hugely by. To put the financial reality of stent procedures into perspective, one quoted cost for a single stent procedure in 2011 was $47,860, with an uninsured discount as a self-pay patient of $19,144, a balance due of

$28,716, and a cardiologist's fee of $2,277. Medicare ended up investigating the Baltimore-area cardiologist and concluded that the situation was simply one of an individual with a problem. Clearly, that one doctor does have a problem, but the self-referral issue is systemic and deeply engrained in American medicine.

Self-referrals form the financial backbone of many specialties. If you walk into an orthopedist's office with back pain, there's a higher chance that you're going to have a surgical procedure than if you had walked into a family doctor's office. Walk into a gastroenterologist's office with stomach pain, and you're more likely to have an expensive diagnostic test or procedure such as endoscopy than if you had walked into a family doctor's office. Fee-for-service reimbursement has created a system where physicians are incentivized to do procedures – and then incentivized to own the equipment they do the procedures on. At the same time they're disincentivized to spend time simply talking with patients, since the amount of money they're paid for patient visits has been decreased. Until those financial incentives and disincentives in the fee-for-service system are reevaluated and restructured, the rest of the healthcare debate is just spitting in the wind. In addition, consumers have been encouraged by the media and by hospital marketing to believe that "high-tech procedures" by definition mean "the best" care, when that's not always the case. High-tech doesn't necessarily mean high value – it sometimes means simply high reimbursement for physicians and hospitals.

Sacred cows: the issue of choice

Physicians and patients aren't alone in putting a premium on the value of choice, of course; Americans as a culture have paid premium dollars for increased choice in every arena of life. Some people with cancer who want to try an experimental drug that their insurance company won't pay for feel they have a right to have the drug covered. But if no one knows whether the drug is going to work, should the rest of society pay for it? There's no easy answer to that, but the question has to stay central to the overall healthcare debate. To what extent is health care a social entitlement versus an individual's responsibility to buy as a consumer product or service?

I would argue that people shouldn't be entitled to insurance company payment for treatment where evidence shows that it probably shouldn't be done. But unproven, experimental treatment, for instance, could be paid for through health savings accounts that allow individuals to set aside a small amount of tax-free income for healthcare costs.

Politicians, when it serves them, spin the choice issue into some variation of the sound bite that "care was denied." A member of Congress from Washington State did that effectively with the child whose mother died of breast cancer; given clinical realities, the mother would have died in any case, but the spin doctors played up the tragedy of a child who's now motherless because the insurer wouldn't pay for care.

There are too many sacred cows in health care; one of them is limitless consumer choice. Another is that whatever a doctor wants or a patient wants, someone else should pay for. All of us are the "someone else"; we're all paying into the system for any unnecessary care through taxes, increased co-pays, and higher co-insurance.

For physicians indoctrinated into a culture of autonomy, if they decide a given treatment is the best option for their patients, they frankly don't want payers questioning that. It had never been questioned – until the advent of insurance and managed care. Many years ago, before insurance, it was only questioned directly by patients. Payment was between patient and doctor with no middlemen, and patients would ask if a treatment was really necessary and negotiate what they could afford to pay. Now the patient isn't paying for the service – at least not directly, and often not the full amount.

Since teasing out the real cost of medical care is impossible when so much is invisible and with so many middlemen and money changing hands, there's a shell game going on, with both cost-shuffling and cost-shifting. Hospitals have undeniable "loss leaders," patient populations requiring long-term care that's poorly reimbursed, such as those with congestive heart failure, and that lost revenue has to be recovered somewhere and balanced out at the end of the year.

So the hospital promotes its cardiac catheterization lab, hoping to shuffle costs by doing more cardiac procedures. Cardiology programs in most hospitals are like the football programs in most universities, which generate the income to pay for field hockey, water polo, and other small programs that lose money every year. Hospitals are forced toward cost-shifting when people without insurance arrive at the hospital and need treatment: Without the benefit of the group purchasing power of large insurers, the uninsured receive astronomical hospital bills. Hospitals hope that enough uninsured people can actually pay their bills, although increasingly that's not the case.

Reevaluating the use of medical technology

One of the potential downsides of healthcare reform is limiting access to new technology, through measures that would encourage waiting to adopt it until adequate data proves that the new technology is truly beneficial. By definition this limits access by limiting the use of technologies that add little or no value; in addition, a regulatory agency would have to oversee a larger budget to investigate new technology benefits. The return on investment for new technology would be much riskier under such a proposal, which is one of the reasons why the United States has led most early adopters; here it's more likely that new technology will be reimbursed earlier and utilized more. Essentially, the healthcare insurance market continues to subsidize medical innovation and research because it's reimbursing doctors and hospitals for most new medical devices and drugs at their costs. But that's not the kind of research currently needed.

The ideal research would integrate the concept of value. Researchers would conduct trials to evaluate which of several different technologies made the biggest difference in long-term health outcomes, given a set amount of money in the national healthcare budget – before deciding whether to advise providers to adopt it universally. If you have a budget you have to manage, you're going to look at new technology much more skeptically, which is what integrated healthcare systems successfully do.

But in the current fee-for-service mentality, everyone's looking for ways to increase revenue to survive. The real question is: What would happen if we discovered, for instance, that we as a society had too many diagnostic imaging machines already? That's a dangerous conversation few physicians and hospital CEOs want to have, because who's going to volunteer to give up their business? As spiraling national costs force the healthcare industry to become more scrutinized, large third-party payers such as Medicare will likely increase their bundling of services and shift more costs to providers. When hospitals begin to receive one check to care for everyone in their geographical area and realize that they have five CT scanners in that area, they're going to ask if they really need to staff all five, how much it actually costs to do each scan, and how many patients actually need the test.

Reframing competing incentives

Medicare currently writes checks to hospitals for bundled services under Medicare Part A payments, but continues to pay for physicians' services under Medicare Part B in the fee-for-service mode. This perpetuates the system of competing incentives between hospitals and the doctors who work there. The hospital is incentivized to spend the bare minimum on patient care, to limit procedures and testing, use the cheapest drugs, and keep the hospital stays short; while the doctor is incentivized to perform procedures, order tests, and increase the number of patient contacts – and has no disincentive not to choose the most expensive drug therapy.

If Medicare were instead to write one bundled check to an integrated healthcare system comprised of hospital services plus physicians' care, including all inpatient and outpatient care for patients with a given disease for a certain number of days, suddenly the incentives of both hospitals and doctors would align. Instead of benefiting financially by doing multiple, repeated CT scans, the incentive would be the opposite:

The team would question how many scans they do and how many CT scanners they really need. They may not need three or four scanners; they may only need one or one-and-a-half staffed scanners and decide to share one with another hospital.

The trend toward a reevaluation of how we use technology will likely push U.S. healthcare patterns closer to those seen in other developed countries rather than continue our current overutilization of CT, MRI, and other technologies. Our country is already hugely oversubscribed with medical imaging technology; you can walk into a shopping mall and have an immediate mammogram or chest x-ray. The contraction in the number of imaging centers, while inevitable, will cause significant future problems for the physicians who own or work in those facilities.

Shifts in pharmaceutical marketing

The relatively new phenomenon of direct-to-consumer marketing is, indirectly, thanks to the work of the late Senator Ted Kennedy, and it's a typical example of how government – even given the best intentions – can make a problem worse by not fully understanding the subtleties of health care. Kennedy believed that the relationship between pharmaceutical companies and doctors looked much too cozy. Pharmaceutical reps were taking physicians to lavish resorts, wining and dining them, showing them their latest drug studies and data – and then, most important – finding out that this kind of high-end marketing to physicians really worked. Doctors went home and ordered their drugs.

Senator Kennedy helped bring the issue of pharmaceutical marketing to consumers' attention through public hearings in 1974 and again in 1990. In fact, the looming 1990 hearings triggered the adoption of stricter guidelines on pharmaceutical marketing and gift-giving to physicians. Shortly before those hearings, the AMA adopted the new guidelines on gift-giving from drug companies as part of their official Code of Ethics. The guidelines stipulate that gifts from drug companies to doctors can't be expensive, can't depend on physicians' prescribing practices or other behavior, and should have the potential of benefiting patients. Further guidelines requested drug companies to disperse financial support for continuing education meetings only to continuing medical education course directors, not to individual physicians.

Later in 1990, the AMA House of Delegates adopted a resolution urging drug companies to limit gifts to those of educational or direct patient benefit, and to use the money thus saved to reduce drug prices. That same year, the American College of Physicians adopted guidelines urging doctors to reject any gifts that might "alter clinical judgment" and to participate only in scientifically sound drug-company sponsored research. Ted Kennedy's hard work stopped the previous, more lavish, physician marketing and put pressure on medical societies to reform. But the reality is that the strategists running the pharmaceutical industry tend to be more sophisticated in how they understand healthcare spending than politicians, who have an inbox full of urgent issues in addition to health care that they must follow. The pharmaceutical strategists reconsidered how they were going to spend those huge annual marketing budgets they had been spending on physicians, and quickly saw an open door to marketing to consumers. Increasingly, companies who make healthcare products of all kinds now market directly to consumers; pharmaceuticals have led the way, spending $5 billion on direct-to-consumer marketing through television and online media.

If you consider the big picture of health care in America, the real question here is: Is it better for drug companies to spend millions of dollars marketing to consumers who have no medically trained filter to be able to sift through what's medically correct, and then have those patients argue with their doctors about what medication he or she suggests? Or is it better to market to physicians, who have the training to recognize when a new drug or drug packaging presented to them is unnecessary, potentially too risky for patients, not really an improvement over what's already available, or even ridiculous?

In the now-insidious, direct-to-consumer TV ads that promote drugs directly to patients, the most untenable part comes at the end, when a woman with an attractive, inviting voice reads off a few of the side effects, which include a few terrible outcomes. How are patients to make any sense of that data? An ad currently running for an asthma drug features a woman's lilting voice that says, "Side effects include unexplained sudden death."

Clearly, the pharmaceuticals' marketing strategists would stop running those ads if they were losing money on them. They've gathered the data to know that enough of those patients go to their doctors and insist on the drug they saw advertised on television – and they know that most doctors don't have time to argue with their patients and don't want to risk losing them, so doctors often agree and prescribe the requested drug. If we as a society decide that we're going to control the marketing of drugs and medical products, it only makes sense to think through the most productive and realistic way to do that.

Unnecessary care: the value of clinical data

Within health care, we need a more cohesive mechanism to question the value of certain kinds of care. Before we decide as a society to adopt certain kinds of screening, for instance, we need to figure out what we're going to do with the information that's uncovered. If you could take a diagnostic test and discover that you have a 60% chance of stroke in the next two years – and you're already exercising, watching your diet, taking the right medications, and not smoking – then what? We have no clinically proven pathways for what to do with that information. It illustrates another problem with the balkanization of medicine: Companies offering a test like that have no skin in the game about what to do with the test results. They're essentially selling consumers useless information and walking away.

The marketing line when selling a test like that to consumers is, "Now that you know about your health risk, you can move into high gear with preventive care, a healthy lifestyle, the right diet and exercise plan to modify or control your risk." But many consumers already know that if they're sedentary and overweight, they smoke and have type 2 diabetes, they're by definition at high risk for stroke, so what real benefit does the test provide? If you find out you have a 60% stenosis and a moderate risk of stroke, what would I, as a cardiologist, tell you? I might check your cholesterol and advise you to exercise more, but you probably know you should be doing that already. While a diagnostic test showing a 60% risk of stroke may be helpful in motivating some patients, its role as a routine test remains unclear.

Clinically, there's a big gap in our knowledge about primary prevention (measures taken to prevent disease, such as before a first-time stroke or heart attack) and secondary prevention (measures taken once disease is present to avert further disease). Clearly, if you've had a stroke before, then the protocol for your care will be more intensive. But as a healthy consumer, simply finding out your risk for a stroke per se, in practical terms, leads to modifying your risk factors, nothing more. So if we're going to spend the money to screen an entire community, we need to decide what to do with the information – and whether it's even valuable. A community decision that everyone over 50 ought to have a given test will prove cost-effective only if we agree what the results actually mean and what to do with them.

Balkanization and variant costs

Reframing the healthcare debate also requires an understanding of how the balkanization of medicine has created widely divergent clinical pathways that lead to wildly variant costs. In most parts of the country, the results of a given diagnostic test lead to different pathways of care, depending on the type of healthcare delivery system that a consumer goes to after the test. Let's say you took the test that indicated you were at risk for a stroke. If you're a member of a prepaid, integrated delivery system such as Group Health in Seattle or Kaiser-Permanente in California and had to pay for the test on your own, your physician would probably check your cholesterol, put you on aspirin, and tell you to exercise.

But if you walk into a vascular surgeon's office with those same test results and you're well covered through private insurance, you could easily end up having a carotid endarterectomy, a surgical procedure to remove the plaque narrowing the artery – two very different clinical decision-making pathways, and two systems that would claim they're doing the right thing for patients and offering the best possible care. Providers in both systems are aware of the same data, but they're interpreting and using the data in very different ways. One system is spending $50 (the cost of the office visit), while the other system is spending money to cover a carotid endarterectomy with a "list price" of over $38,000, a price for consumers with insurance of over $17,000, and a typical patient's out-of-pocket expense of close to $1,000.

That's a prime example of the question of value in health care. Where is the value in each different pathway? Have our country's clinical research teams provided the outcomes research and medical evidence to determine which pathways are most likely to lead to the best long-term outcomes? The fact is that, for the overwhelming number of diseases, they haven't.

Evidence-based medicine is still in its embryonic stage. Of all the things we physicians do, there's a relatively small body of knowledge where it's absolutely clear-cut what the best treatment protocol is. That body of knowledge continues to expand as we improve our informatics to be able to share data across various hospital, provider, and payer systems. But the judgment of physicians and the art of medicine will never disappear. Medicine isn't nuclear physics; it isn't an exact science and never will be. Developing the art of evidence-based clinical pathways is a key arena in which physician leaders can have a huge impact on value-driven health care in the future.

Creating a value analysis on new technology

In the absence of a comprehensive body of outcomes research, how do we make decisions about what to do with the data we do have, when there is no one, right answer based on conclusive studies? One promising solution is through integrated healthcare delivery systems. If both a primary care physician and an independent vascular surgeon were in the same integrated healthcare delivery system, both with a clinical point of view and trying to do the best thing for the patient, the surgeon would have to justify spending 40 times as much – knowing that spending 40 times as much means there's less money to provide other care in that system.

This may be a different way for some American physicians to think about what they do: keeping the big picture in mind. That's what's missing. Physicians in Canada, England, and Germany all want to do what's best for their patients, too, but they're forced to come to grips with the reality that they have to justify how they're spending their healthcare system's dollars by advising certain treatment options.

In our country, when a new technology becomes available, perhaps we need a separate budget to evaluate it, look at it objectively, and compare it to other current options. We're now paying for technology based on what it cost the manufacturer to produce, including their profit margins – not on its real value. Medical technology is exploding because it's so rich in profit opportunities; whatever medical device companies produce, our healthcare system pays for it, including development costs. Typically, new medical device development is funded directly within large, already successful companies or through start-ups later acquired by those large companies. Their return on investment comes from a market where our government or insurance companies are likely to reimburse well for the technology.

The lack of a solid lid on healthcare spending has created a huge market opportunity for these medical technology players. It's a high-stakes game, so when negative data is published, the developers argue that those poor outcomes were based on an older version of the technology, and they go back to the drawing board to develop a new, "improved" version.

When several randomized trials showed, for instance, that elective coronary stenting does not, in fact, reduce the incidence of heart attacks or prolong life, it was depressing news to the investors in the stent company and the cardiologists making their living doing stents.

So after the negative studies were published, the physicians who were making their clinical or academic careers doing stents wrote back to the editorial page of the medical journals that had published the studies. They argued that the randomized trials had several flaws and that those patients were all given bare-metal stents instead of the newer, drug-eluting stents; therefore, the negative data was irrelevant. I suspect, when future data shows that the drug-eluting stents have no real benefit, either, that their new counter-argument will be that they were using the wrong medication and the new drug-eluting stents use a new, "improved" drug.

The same phenomenon occurred with bypass surgery, which I saw first-hand while involved with some of the original research as a Cardiovascular Fellow at the University of Washington in Seattle in 1979. Researchers found that except for a small subset of patients – those with disease in the left main coronary artery – bypass surgery didn't seem to make any difference in survival in patients with coronary artery disease.

Researchers did further analysis and found that if a patient had left main artery disease or severe three-vessel disease and poor ventricular function – in others words, a severe amount of heart damage and three-vessel disease – bypass surgery may help. But in all the other patients – the majority of patients – it didn't seem to make any difference. Yet every time those negative articles were published showing no real benefit to the majority of patients undergoing bypass surgery, cardiac surgeons argued that the studies didn't yet use some newer drug, or used the wrong technique, or used veins instead of arteries, and on and on. The data is ignored; it's rationalized away. In a practical sense, it's understandable: If a cardiac surgeon trained for seven years of his or her life to do bypass surgery or a cardiologist trained for four or five years to place stents, and later research discovered that those procedures were ineffective, that surgeon or cardiologist is likely to go on the defensive and come up with counter-arguments. The bottom line? Our country ends up with an unhealthy system where physicians argue against the data while continuing to be well paid for procedures that may have no real benefit.

The confusion and cost to the system are especially noticeable with the high-ticket, high-tech items that hospitals promote. If a hospital begins marketing 3D mammography as a better test and "the next big thing," consumers, who already believe that mammography is worthwhile for the early detection of breast cancer, are likely to request it – even though it's unproven. By definition, when a new technology comes along and receives reimbursement, there's not going to be a lot of data on it. The need for unbiased data and big-picture thinking are central to the healthcare debate, so that providers and the public alike can benefit from analysis not driven by special interests of the financial "winners" in the system.

A single-party payer, market competition, and value

With a single-party-payer system, a country's government makes a decision about how much money to spend on health care each year as a percentage of GDP. Depending on the size of the country, funds are either administered through a centralized agency or through smaller states or provinces. The Canadian model is a case in point; each province receives a budget and has a committee of bureaucrats who decide how it's going to be spent. Each hospital and community submits a requested budget, they fight back and forth with the government to hammer it out, and that's what there is to spend. Hospitals and physicians have separate budgets, with physicians as government employees who bill the provincial government on a fixed fee-for-service basis. When they run out of money, that's it, except for a few emergency situations. Obviously, they're not going to let people bleed to death, but they do queue up cases that aren't emergencies into the next year's budget.

In reality, many Canadians who can afford it come to the United States for health care when it's denied them or postponed too long in Canada. Through its political system, Canada at times creates a supplemental budget where they don't give the money to a province but instead contract with a U.S. healthcare organization to provide certain "emergency" services. Through the 1980s and 1990s when I was practicing, our cardiology practice in Seattle and the hospital where we practiced both received checks from the Canadian government from time to time to provide cardiac services for Canadians from British Columbia who were too far down on the list and couldn't get in for treatment during that budget year. Canada has contracted with American hospitals to perform angioplasties for heart disease, bone marrow transplants for cancer, bariatric surgery for obesity, diagnostic imaging tests, and other services not readily available in their own healthcare system.

There's no question that if you need a hip replacement in Canada, you're going to wait a lot longer than you will in the States, and if you need certain diagnostic procedures, you're going to have to travel much further for them. There are certainly people in Canada who are frustrated with the inconvenience, the lines, and the waiting, though the magnitude of the wait depends on when they need treatment within the budgetary process. The wait lines tend to be fairly short early on in their fiscal year, but as they're running out of money, the wait is longer. You can get a hip replacement within a day or two in the States, and people can wait months or longer in Canada. A lot depends on the patient's age, severity of the problem, and other factors that go into the Canadian queue, although personal income isn't a factor. Canadians can't buy their way to the top of the queue, but they can buy their way into the United States for surgery.

Understanding physician resistance to a single-party payer

The single-party-payer concept has a rich history in our country, one that sheds light on the current debate. Harry Truman and other presidents tried to bring national health care to the United States via a single-party payer along the lines of other developed countries. But when physicians hear any talk of national health care, they see a loss of autonomy and being controlled by bureaucrats who don't necessarily understand the nuances of health care. They fear seeing their patients waiting for procedures instead of being able to have them when they need them. They fear stagnation in new medical technologies, with the innovation that they've taken for granted in this country brought to a grinding halt.

An even larger fear surrounds the loss of income. Physicians in many countries with national health care earn considerably less income than physicians in the United States. In Israel, for instance, with socialized medicine, physicians earn the equivalent of US$ 66,000 a year. The Israel Medical Association recently requested a large salary increase for doctors so that the average wage for a physician in a state-owned hospital would rise from NIS (Israeli new shekel) 20,191 a month in gross wages to NIS 26,813. To put that income into perspective, Israeli doctors' salaries are comparable to what Israeli school teachers or construction workers earn; they're certainly not an elite part of society as physicians are today in the United States. Granted, that may be an extreme example; Canadian physicians earn less than American physicians, but they're still earning upper-middle-class incomes of up to a couple hundred thousand dollars a year.

The fear among American physicians lies not only in having their incomes severely cut with the initiation of any form of single-party-payer system; it's also that they'll have no control over their future incomes. They fear that once a central bureaucracy starts making decisions about clinical care and medical budgets, that same bureaucracy could arbitrarily start paying doctors whatever they decide. But doctors don't see themselves as members of a union now and don't welcome the idea of being members of a union in the future. Physicians see themselves as autonomous professionals, not as collective bargainers, and many of them have a healthy fear of the government running health care; the track record given Medicare and Medicaid is spotty. Doctors are smart enough to worry that the government will control their livelihood and incomes once it starts fixing their rates.

Physicians also fear an overall decrease in the quality of health care with a single-party payer. Along with stagnation in innovation, they're worried that new doctors won't be attracted into medicine because of fixed pay, increased bureaucratic oversight, and loss of autonomy. If their income drops, doctors also worry that they're not going to have control over their office staffs due to limitations on what they can afford to pay people, and that they won't be able to attract the quality of staff they can attract now. Office nurses today tend to be very bright and make good incomes. Doctors, especially in primary care, may not be able to afford that kind of help in the future, and they may have restrictions on how their office staff works; their staff may, in fact, work for the government.

All of these legitimate reasons make doctors leery of a single-party payer, but it's critical to remember that physicians are not a homogenous community. Some physicians would welcome a single-party payer, particularly those in specialties who are getting squeezed now and would likely benefit financially by the change. Primary care doctors, in general, accept the idea more than specialists, no doubt due to the huge discrepancy in incomes between primary and specialty care physicians. Some primary care doctors in Seattle, for instance, earn less than $100,000 a year, while it's not unusual for some specialists to earn more than $1 million a year. Different specialists and types of physician groups see the pros and cons of a single-party-payer system through their own unique lenses, with a greater or lesser resistance to the changes they'd be forced to make in how they practice medicine.

Rather than a single-party payer, then, our country could end up with a handful of competing healthcare systems, all incentivized to compete on quality, cost, or both – to compete on value. There may be good clinical reasons, for instance, to provide a given screening test to people, and the system that offers it may attract consumers who see that as a value proposition. In general, societies that have relied on central planning haven't done as well in terms of overall national health; better decisions are typically made on a community level so that local populations' needs can be addressed.

Sound bite: "cherry-picking"

The "Harry and Louise" sound bites during former president Bill Clinton's era, sponsored by the insurance industry, claimed that Clinton wanted to have bureaucrats replace doctors in decision-making, which was not exactly what the healthcare reform plan had in mind. But it worked as a scare tactic. Years later, in the debate between Barack Obama and Hillary Clinton during the 2008 presidential primary, the fundamental difference between their views on health care was that Hillary Clinton wanted to mandate that everyone had to have insurance and not allow an option out. Obama wanted people to have a choice.

This cuts to the issue of "cherry picking" in the insurance industry. The dilemma is that if you don't require everyone to have insurance, people without insurance have a hard time affording it. The insurance companies, without any kind of regulation, will go out of their way to insure people who are least likely to use insurance – and then charge higher premiums to those likely to need it.

Most insurance works by rating your premiums based on your medical risks and the potential cost to the insurer to cover you. Clearly, it costs them a lot more money to cover older people and those with chronic conditions requiring lifelong care. So the debate with reform is how to force insurance companies to take on everyone – for instance, not allow them to charge more for preexisting conditions but instead offer the same rates for everyone. If you insure everyone and insist that you can't deny insurance, can't "rate" people, and can't price insurance higher for people at higher risk, what you have to do as an insurer to survive is to pass that cost on to people who are at less risk. That may be something that society decides to accept, but it would mean that keeping current insurance plans without changing anything is a fallacy. The illusion of unlimited access and choice without increasing costs simply doesn't bear scrutiny.

Market forces are a reality in health care. Insurance companies have to make a profit and report to their shareholders, and they currently make profits by preferentially offering insurance at lower rates to people who are unlikely to use it. If you regulate the industry and prevent them from doing this, you'll create huge resistance – and lobbying efforts – from the entire industry.

Managed care in the 1980s brought on the era of an explosion of choice: consumers "doctor shopping" and frequently switching policies from one insurance plan and primary care doctor one year to new ones the next. The response in the physician community has been a degree of resignation, knowing that it's not the ideal way to provide care, but accommodating themselves to it after the rise of managed care plans. Most physician groups in a given community are now affiliated with most local health plans – which, ironically, have rarely been able to negotiate large cost savings because they're locked into the dysfunctional fee-for-service mode based on physicians' historical professional fees and technical fees. Without shifting the fee-for-service mindset, the chess game is still the same, and the healthcare crisis isn't going to change.

When a private insurer negotiates with all the cardiologists in Seattle, for instance, to determine professional fees for cardiac catheterization, the degree of negotiation between insurance companies and physicians depends on the size of the physician group. The smaller the group, the less leverage it has in negotiating with insurers; but it's shaped by the size and clout of the insurers' market share as well. If an insurer that controlled 30% of the market came in and said they'd pay cardiologists $1,500 to do a stent procedure when the going rate all along had been $2,000, the cardiologists would have to think twice about not signing up. To a certain extent, the market drives how flexible physicians can be and stay competitive. But since health care is not a typical commodity, those market rules have a limited effect in controlling overall costs.

Chapter 4
The Crisis in the Physician Community

In August 2010, when I moderated the meeting of Washington State's Eighth Congressional District Health Care Advisory Board with Representative Dave Reichert, I asked each leader present from a local healthcare organization to report in and then address the critical issue of how to fix our national healthcare system. Reichert, who sits on the Congressional Ways and Means Committee, wanted our regional input on the sustainable growth rate (SGR), a formula in Medicare that reduces physician reimbursement yearly whenever Medicare spending outpaces our country's gross domestic product.

Congress has waived the SGR nearly every year since its inception but has not repealed it, so the SGR hangs over physicians' heads each year. As of December 2011, when Congress sat in stalemate over reducing Medicare payments to doctors, doctors faced a 27% cut in their payments from Medicare to begin in January 2012; legislation then postponed the cuts until March 2012. These payment cuts, planned as percentage cuts across the board, continue to hurt primary care doctors more than procedural specialty care, since primary care margins are so low to begin with.

In that regional meeting with local hospitals, physicians' groups, and insurers, most of the major healthcare players in the Seattle region agreed that the sustainable growth rate formula isn't working to bring the lowest physician payments up to par, and in fact the whole idea needs to be scrapped. Even more interesting was the general consensus that the fee-for-service system is no longer sustainable. Even the interventional cardiologist at the meeting – a procedure-based specialty typically highly rewarded by fee-for-service payments – didn't protest at that. The times are changing.

Financial uncertainty tops the list of issues driving the crisis in the physician community today. Not only do my physician colleagues agree that the fee-for-service system is disappearing, none of them think that the current system is sustainable even for 20 years. Medicare is not sustainable now. Every time Medicare gives a little more to one specialty for a service, it cuts from another to balance it, but the whole reimbursement system is never balanced in a sensible, workable way. Every time Medicare approves expensive new technology for reimbursement, the funding has to come from somewhere, and with the mandate to use the sustainable growth rate formula for a balanced federal budget, that "somewhere" typically means a reduction in physician reimbursement.

Fading fee-for-service

At the end of that August 2010 Health Care Advisory Board meeting, I broached the subject of prospective payments for care and asked, "Suppose King County had five designated healthcare systems that consumers could pick from, and that system would receive a check for the care of each consumer for one year, allowing that system to figure out how to take care of that patient cost-effectively?" The discussion was illuminating. One objection was that it wouldn't work because not all doctors are employed, but integration has little to do with the structure of physician employment. Another physician thought that prospective payment implied the model of a nonprofit healthcare system that coordinates both care and insurance coverage. The insurance representative said that his company would love to pay prospectively like that, and so did the leaders from a successful, physician-run hospital.

At the end of the day, most providers agreed they'd be much better off managing healthcare dollars than bureaucrats, and the more far-sighted among them have begun novel projects to do just that. The VP of Medical Affairs of a large hospital at the meeting reported that their facility was extending more cost-effective patient care into the community with a trial program where physicians work more in a supervisory capacity, training other caregivers to go to patients' homes and provide the basic care that helps patients stay at home and stay out of the hospital. Their goal is value: to use providers performing at the peak of what they're trained to do – but not more, and not overutilizing their expertise. Using doctors to do home visits, for instance, wouldn't be an efficient, cost-effective use of physician time; someone whose salary reflects less sophisticated training could instead perform many of the home visit tasks. Physicians in this country are an expensively trained, scarce resource, and whatever form reimbursement takes in the future, American doctors should be fairly compensated for their education, skills, and responsibilities.

So while that hospital isn't yet getting reimbursed for that new program, they're still investing in it in anticipation of the current reimbursement system imploding. Most providers are beginning to agree that fee-for-service is dying out and that some form of payment capitation – where a delivery system is paid a set fee to care for each patient per year – will replace it.

Ratcheting down reimbursement

The financial rewards of medicine are difficult to discuss in the healthcare debate, in part because to some people, the definition of someone who "makes too much money" is someone who "makes more money than me." It's challenging for those who are working hard and making $50,000 or $60,000 a year to listen to physicians complain about their reimbursement when the average physician earns $200,000.

But when the country decides to control costs by reducing physician reimbursement, what happens? Decreased reimbursement means it becomes almost impossible for primary care doctors to function as solo practitioners who need to pay their own staffs, rents, and utilities. As Medicare, Medicaid, and private insurers continue to ratchet down how much they pay primary care doctors per patient for office visits, and at the same time physicians' practice overhead costs continue to rise, what are their options? While they're taking home less money, they have to see more patients to avoid going out of business completely, so the patient experience goes way down.

Ratcheting down physician reimbursement on primary care has essentially caused the disappearance of "Dr. Welby," the solo family doctor. Most primary care doctors practice in groups now, often in very large groups. The overhead requirements of a single-office practice have simply become too onerous. Not only do rent, heat, light, and staff salaries go up, now they must add overhead costs to deal with the regulatory environment as it keeps ratcheting up. Doctors either have to hire someone to deal with the regulatory environment and the paperwork for them or spend time away from their patients to deal with it themselves.

Because specialists have a better baseline income and the ability to perform procedures with high reimbursements, they can tolerate today's ratcheting down of reimbursement a bit better. While cardiologists are now reimbursed less to do typical procedures – what used to be a $3,000 procedure might suddenly pay only $2,000 – it still pays better than a typical $50 primary care office visit.

According to the Medical Group Management Association as reported in *Time* magazine in August 2010, primary care doctors earned a median salary of just over $191,000 in 2009. But this number includes money earned through the utilization of doctor-owned (or, in the physician employment model, hospital-owned) laboratories, imaging centers, and surgical facilities. Health reforms in the Affordable Care Act legislation of 2010 added a potential 10% bonus to primary care doctors' reimbursement for Medicare patient visits, but the president of the American Academy of Family Practice has gone on record saying that a 30% to 50% increase is needed to keep primary care afloat and for the system to work.

Every year brings incredible stress for physicians because they have no idea what the percentage drop in their reimbursements will be. Physician payment for procedures and office visits can drop 10%, 20%, 30% or more at a time; payments might then stay the same for a year or two or drop again. The SGR (sustainable growth rate) payment change suggested for 2012 was a 27% drop. How many other professions have borne similar, unpredictable, repeated cuts in pay? Physicians who are self-employed have no long-term contract, so their long-term financial planning becomes an art form at best.

When payment for procedures and office visits drops by 40%, physicians have no redress with the government agencies that cut them. Medicare and Medicaid essentially decide what they're going to pay, and physicians have the option of playing or not playing. Given the size of Medicare, most physicians have no choice but to play. Physicians can't negotiate with Medicare, and private insurers typically follow Medicare. If Medicare gets away with doing something, private insurers end up following suit.

Private insurers often negotiate fees with physicians based on a percentage of Medicare payment; for example, paying 110% of Medicare rates. In one year, urologists were cut nearly 30% across the board for their services. Another year, for cardiologists, electrophysiology and pacemaker procedures were cut. It seems capricious; physicians never know what to expect. It triggers fear and trying to cover for an unknown future, as well as creating a culture of cynicism, dissatisfaction, resignation, and an erosion of the highest values of medicine. When physicians could charge what they thought were reasonable rates and received increases in rates to compete with inflation, their attitude was much different. Now in the era of deep cuts in reimbursement, the risk of the fee-for-service model is its increased potential to stimulate temptation in procedure-based practices, encouraging doctors to sift through patients to "find the gold" of procedures.

Income disparity: primary and specialty care

Turf wars among physicians trying to survive financially take center stage in the interface between primary care doctors and hospitals. Medicare now reimburses primary care doctors little to see patients. A half-hour visit with a patient who has diabetes, congestive heart failure, headache, or depression typically pays a primary care doctor only one-third the amount that a specialist would be paid to perform a diagnostic, surgical, or imaging procedure on that same patient.

The median income of specialists in 2004 was almost twice that of primary care physicians, a gap that is widening. Data from the Medical Group Management Association indicate that from 1995 to 2004, the median income for primary care physicians increased by 21.4%, while that for specialists increased by 37.5%. In 2006 the Center for Studying Health System Change reported that from 1995 to 2003, inflation-adjusted income *decreased* for all physicians by 7.1% and by 10.2% for primary care physicians. When a primary care doctor's patients need to go to the hospital, a specialist sees them and takes over their care, and Medicare only pays the specialist; they won't pay the primary care doctor to provide care during that hospitalization. Beginning in the 1990s, primary care doctors were no longer able to survive by driving to the hospital to spend time checking up on their patients who had been admitted.

The economic squeeze: regulatory time cost

The economic squeeze on physicians grows tighter each year due to increased time demanded by too many regulatory requirements, which takes away from their time with patients. All the additional administrative time, providing extra documentation for services denied by insurers, staying up-to-date on never-ending changes to coding requirements, revising office practices to remain compliant with HIPAA (the

Health Insurance Portability and Accountability Act) and other federal regulations, and performing drug reconciliations and discharge summaries for hospitals are tasks physicians perform gratis.

In fact, the regulatory arena closely scrutinizes any monetary arrangement between hospitals and physicians. It's against the law for hospitals to pay physicians for much of the work that the regulatory environment creates. In that sense, the regulatory environment currently limits the creation of truly integrated healthcare delivery systems where financial incentives of doctors and hospitals align. Even if hospitals had the money to pay physicians for the required regulatory work – and most of them don't – they're not allowed to. It could be construed as a "kick-back" for patient referrals, due to the work of Congressman Pete Stark (D-CA), chairman of the Ways and Means Health Subcommittee from 2007 to 2010, who had raised concerns about the physician-hospital relationship for years.

In fact, in California, hospitals aren't allowed to employ physicians at all, so providers have created large physician foundations with a common board of directors with the hospital, essentially creating hospital subsidiaries. The relationship between physicians and hospitals has long been highly scrutinized, highly regulated, and nearly impossible for any individual hospital to change, even if it might ultimately make good sense for hospitals to pay physicians for the work they do to maintain the hospitals' regulatory and financial responsibilities.

Forced volume

When insurers manage to pay physicians a lot less, what happens? Doctors try to make it up in volume to maintain their profitability. Whether "volume" means doing more cardiac catheterizations or seeing more patients, neither tactic improves overall health care.

Given the recent lowering of reimbursement for primary care doctors, they've been slugging it out in the trenches, seeing 50 or 60 patients a day. But what's the quality of that experience for patients? The patient experience is bound to plummet. How much money is ultimately wasted in the system by medical problems that aren't picked up in those six-minute patient visits, or they're picked up and referred out to expensive specialists because primary care doctors don't have time to deal with them? It's a systemic challenge that physicians could collaborate on solving, working together to design algorithms that coordinate primary and specialty care more effectively. Consumers would benefit in other ways, as well, because the patient experience currently can be terribly frustrating, with patients often spending much more time making the appointment, driving there, and sitting in the waiting room than they do face-to-face with a doctor in the appointment itself. Simply cutting reimbursement further is not the solution, especially with primary care doctors, who'd be forced to spend even less time with each patient.

The overall, long-term consequences for our country's healthcare system with deeper cuts in physician reimbursement also bear considering. Again, national healthcare costs are driven by physician utilization, not by professional compensation. That's why hospitals spend huge amounts of money building state-of-the-art facilities with high-tech diagnostic labs and the latest surgical suite technology. Unfortunately, they end up costing the entire healthcare system a lot more money, with no demonstrable increase in value.

Medical school debt

The paradigm is also shifting because the doctors coming out of training now come out with huge debt. Many opt for employment-type models because they don't want financial uncertainty; they need to receive a regular paycheck to pay down their debt. Increasingly, young doctors trying to balance career and family are less interested in the long hours and lack of a family life that characterized older generations of physicians. The unprecedented debt after medical school is due in large part to medical school costs rising and a big shift out of the public sector in financing medical school tuition. I went to a state-subsidized medical school from 1972 to 1975 and paid $10,800 in tuition. My wife went to an Ivy League medical school, graduating in 1981, and her medical tuition bill was about $100,000.

Among today's graduating medical students, 85% carry outstanding loans. The American Medical Association reports that the average educational debt of medical school graduates in the class of 2010 was $157,944; 78% of graduates had debt of at least $100,000, with 42% carrying at least $150,000. While several medical bloggers believe those figures to be underestimated, clearly the percentage of medical students' personal budgets required every month to pay off medical school debt is high and limits their options regarding where and how they practice.

According to the American Academy of Family Physicians, primary care physicians fare even worse. Its novice physicians carry, on average, $200,000 in loans, and with undergraduate loans and deferred compensation during training, that number can reach well above $500,000. New physicians starting their professional lives with high debt loads clearly face a largely chaotic, uncertain reimbursement environment. Many medical school graduates now look for salaried positions so they can predict their income each year and put aside a portion of that to pay off their debt, as well as buy a house and start a family. They also opt out of primary care; in 2010, only 4.9% of current medical students were heading toward family practice, with less than 2% of students interested in general internal medicine, according to a study published in the *Journal of the American Medical Association*. Why is general internal medicine doing even worse than primary care? Primary care doctors are trained in procedures that can supplement their low patient-care reimbursements with office procedures such as vasectomies, proctoscopies, and skin biopsies.

The physician shortage

The shortage of primary care doctors in the future appears likely to worsen. There won't be enough doctors overall 10 years from now, but the deepest shortfall will come in primary care. The bigger problem will be the lack of any kind of rational distribution of doctors. It's already extremely difficult for physicians to practice in smaller communities, especially in rural environments, based on how reimbursements are paid.

New layers of regulatory requirements are forcing doctors to merge into larger groups to create some kind of economy of scale in dealing with those regulations. A group of 15 or 20 doctors can afford to pay a staffperson to do nothing but deal with the regulatory environment and paperwork, whereas the cost of that person for one physician is prohibitive. A solo practice still needs that staff but doesn't have other doctors with which to share the overhead.

Smaller communities need only one or two doctors, but the problem is finding someone to take that on. A solo doctor never gets a day off and is bound to have some patients who simply can't afford to pay. Some of the difficulties of luring physicians into rural practice may be eased by technology down the road, but it's been a huge problem for years and is likely to become worse.

With demographics shifting toward baby boomers, many of whom will have age-related chronic disease, the system will need more physicians taking care of them, but we're not expanding medical schools to address that. In addition, physician burnout drives a lot of doctors out of medicine toward other careers or early retirement, and that creates gaps. More and more doctors are retiring earlier.

In addition, young doctors training now are indoctrinated with new expectations in terms of how many hours they'll work. If the average physician now works 60 hours a week and future doctors will be working only 40 hours a week, we're going to need more docs. Based on our current reimbursement system, it's a given. It's possible, if we changed the reimbursement system and became more efficient in using doctors, then we wouldn't need as many; but physician time management and utilization hasn't yet been studied in a systematic way. Physician training is extremely expensive and hard to sustain, especially at the postgraduate level, so it's unlikely we'll see a burst of new medical schools opening in the near term. Roughly half of all medical students now are women, so in 10 or 15 years half of all physicians in practice will be women. Many of them elect to practice part-time, another factor to consider when it comes to calculating the nation's need for fulltime physicians.

If a significant percentage of female medical school graduates decide they're not going to work fulltime, the system has even fewer trained physicians to do the work of one fulltime employee. A *New York Times* op-ed piece in 2011 referenced the American Academy of Pediatrics estimate that over 70% of female pediatricians take extended leaves from practice, five times more than the percentage of male pediatricians. If it takes two female graduates to cover one fulltime position, or four new physicians to cover five fulltime positions – and we already have a shortage of fulltime physicians – it exaggerates the problem.

Shifting costs and decisions to consumers

Multiple changes are set in motion as more healthcare costs are shifted directly to the consumer's pocketbook. In the past, when patients paid a $10 co-pay out-of-pocket for a bypass surgery or hip replacement, they didn't think too long or hard about which hospital they were going to and who was doing the surgery. They didn't have much skin in the game at all.

Now, as consumers are paying much more through higher co-pays and deductibles, they're evaluating that care much more carefully. If they're spending $10,000 out-of-pocket for surgery, they want more information. They're going to sources other than their friends and the local hospital, such as HealthGrades and other online content and rating sources, to try to make a good decision about their care. Unfortunately, the data available today on hospital and physician "outcomes" is incomplete and fragmented, making those online sources unreliable. Consumers won't be able to find the kind of information that will be truly useful until value is created in health care.

Many people receive information about health care from doctors or people they trust who have recently received similar care. Internet surfing may replace this method, but it, too, is based largely on subjective experience. A site like Angie's List may be a good place to find a plumber, where the value proposition is easy to measure: "He showed up, didn't rob me, fixed my sink, and cleaned up afterwards." With health care, more complex realities abound, and unfortunately, many patients undergo unnecessary procedures and are still convinced that their doctor saved their lives. The focus on "the patient's experience" may enhance family, friend, and online referrals, but it won't change the high rate of unnecessary procedures or unnecessary utilization. It's not going to change the dynamic of how much time a physician can spend with a patient, although it may help the flow of patients through the system so they can be seen more quickly on a regular basis. Patients typically go to those "patient-centric" facilities not because they offer better quality care but because they're convenient.

Even as a physician in a better-than-average position to judge quality of care, I tend to choose a regional healthcare system where I can make an appointment quickly, get in quickly, and not be kept waiting when I arrive. Physicians in a system like that are very much aware of the patient experience they're offering; and while I applaud those efforts, it's not going to lower healthcare costs. Simple economics can't be ignored: Once physicians and hospitals start earning less per product or service, the only way they're going to stay afloat, under our current dysfunctional reimbursement system, is to produce lower-quality services or produce more of them.

New paradigms outpace training

Young physicians are still taught in the traditional mode, with physicians primarily trained to be autonomous. But without enough initial selection or later training on how to be effective, collaborative leaders, young physicians leave their training programs unprepared for what's happening in practice. The new paradigms are outpacing training: Medical students aren't developing the skills they need to work well and communicate well as part of a team. In the last few years, medical schools are beginning to incorporate some "real world" truths in training, but in general, training programs are insulated from many of the realities of private practice and working in busy community hospitals. The academic tradition of medicine, both among its faculty and in its training, doesn't always adapt quickly as culture changes.

The medical school experience has radically changed from the era of the exhausted med student forced to do endless shifts in a row. The new regulatory environment that controls training has created an "easier" culture: Interns and residents now have limited hours they're allowed to work, and once they put in their hours, they're not allowed to stay in the hospital. On the one hand, that's a positive thing, since interns and residents can make mistakes and become cranky when they're exhausted. On the other hand, it creates a mindset that doesn't match the reality of practice. Medicine is not an eight-to-five job. I often speak with young med students and new graduates, and their expectations about how hard they're going to work is very different from when my generation went through medical training. We expected to work around the clock in our medical training, and most of us carried that expectation of long hours and incredibly hard work into practice.

I had "no life" during the three years of my internal medicine training and little in the way of a life during my fellowship. For our ICU rotation, we were on-call every other night. We didn't leave the hospital for the night we were "off" until all of our work was completed and we could sign off with the next physician coming on-call. The nights we were "off," if we were out of the hospital by 8:00 PM we were doing well. Throughout my career, when I was on-call as a practicing physician, I was immediately available to my patients and didn't put myself in situations where I couldn't be responsible and act quickly. My generation of physicians has a hard time imagining what medicine will be like with an eight-to-five mindset and practice. How will Americans adjust to the idea of going into a physician's office like a gas station, with different attendants for different shifts? That's vastly different from how most of us began our professional lives, with a vastly different level of commitment to our patients. The gap now being created between medical students' expectations in school and what they're going to face when they enter practice further demoralizes the physician community.

Medical schools also still train physicians based on an old paradigm: Doctors are the repository of all relevant information, and they're in charge. But that's no longer the way it is –not in the office and certainly not in the hospital. The old paradigm of this kind of "leadership" needs to be replaced with a new paradigm of true leadership to boost morale in the physician community. Too many physicians are completely burned out, walking around with their heads down all day, feeling trapped. They're working 60 to 80 hours a week, spending more and more time each year on regulatory documentation and not patient care. There's a lack of optimism about the future.

The Willie Sutton principle: high-yield activities

The unaddressed issue playing out in the dysfunctional reimbursement scheme – the question we as a society must answer – is deciding the "fair market value" for doctors' services and how to determine that. Another way to look at physicians' professional fees is to ask: Are doctors as valuable as lawyers? As CEOs of small businesses? We could compare other professional salaries to physicians' salaries to arrive at a range that's reasonable for doctors' level of education and training. Creating a system in which physicians are reimbursed based on fair market value would eliminate a lot of other issues, such as the financial incentives for overutilization.

Consumers have been led to believe that high physician salaries are the problem, but in fact physicians' "professional fees" are a drop in the bucket of overall healthcare costs compared to "facility fees" and "technical fees," some of which are for unnecessary procedures. This is a leap-of-faith argument, though, since there's currently no accurate way to evaluate all procedures performed and determine how many of them were unnecessary. Actuaries make estimates all the time, but estimates are just guesses.

Willie Sutton, the notorious bank robber, was once asked why he chose to rob banks. "That's where the money is," he replied. In health care, it's clear that the push toward the Willie Sutton principle – the focus on high-yield activities – such as when physicians own their own diagnostic equipment and surgical centers, is a dangerous and costly direction for medicine. When physicians were making incomes they were satisfied with, there wasn't a problem; they could go into medicine to take care of patients, knowing they'd be fairly compensated for their efforts.

It's telling that, increasingly, when physicians are interviewed, they say they don't want their children going into medicine; they would not recommend it as a career. Traditionally, physicians have had high divorce rates since it's challenging to be married to a busy doctor. The hours, the stress, the responsibility – even before issues with reimbursement, many physicians tend to think constantly about patients they saw that day and what they could have done better. We're seldom home, and when we are home, we're wearing a beeper, or we're on the phone. It wasn't so long ago that physicians wanted their kids to go into medicine with them; many doctors dreamed of having one of their children practicing with them. Very few docs say that anymore. When you ask them whether things will get better or worse in the next five to 10 years, they all uniformly say they're going to get worse.

That's part of the incredible phenomenon going on right now: Physicians feel they're losing all their autonomy, they're not being valued or heard, and there's a sense of victimization in the physician culture.

Turf wars among specialties

The current competitive environment among different kinds of physicians adds to the low morale. A prime example: A relatively new technology, yet to be scientifically proven in terms of its value relative to morbidity and mortality, is placing stents in peripheral arteries to treat peripheral vascular disease or renal artery stenosis (narrowing of the arteries that carry blood to the kidneys) as opposed to surgery.

Regardless of the lack of data supporting long-term clinical effectiveness, it's fairly well reimbursed and seems an attractive alternative to peripheral bypass surgery.

But in today's competitive medical environment, the question isn't "what's the value?" but "who gets to do it?" The radiologists argue that their expertise lies in injecting contrast dyes into arteries everywhere in the body, so they ought to do it. The cardiologists argue that they can put a stent in a 2.5 mm artery in heart muscle that's constantly moving, and safely inject dye into the coronary arteries in a procedure that carries the risk of arrhythmia and sudden death, so they're certainly the most qualified to put a simple stent in a leg that's not moving at all, with an easy-to-visualize artery 10 times larger than the coronary artery and with no risk of sudden death during the procedure; so they should do it. The vascular surgeons argue that only they should be allowed to do the procedure, since they spent four or five years of their professional lives focused solely on vascular disease and vascular surgery, and, unlike cardiologists or radiologists, they're trained to handle stent complications requiring surgery.

Who wins? Hospitals try to avoid the battle by forming committees and trying to delay the decision; but when push comes to shove, if cardiologists want to do a new procedure, they're going to do it. Ultimately, it's a political decision within the hospital, driven by healthcare economics and based on revenue. Cardiologists bring countless patients into the hospital – a high volume of patients who are profitable for the hospital, due in large part to their high number of profitable procedures. Vascular surgeons bring in fewer patients, and the hospital loses money on a lot of them. The radiologists bring in no patients; they're dependent on the hospital for their business, so they have no political clout. Likewise, the hospital traditionally has been the referral source for intravascular radiologists, so if an intravascular radiologist quits, the hospital just hires a new one.

The cost of malpractice insurance

Consumers may have heard that one of the major reasons doctors are going out of business is the high cost of their malpractice insurance, but the truth is, it depends on the specialty. The facts are a lot more nuanced than the sound bites. Certain specialties have been clobbered by malpractice insurance. One of them is obstetrics, where many Ob-Gyn docs are giving up obstetrics because their malpractice insurance is so expensive they can't afford it; they end up practicing only gynecology. Malpractice insurance has also had an impact in terms of physician migration since malpractice insurance rates are set by each state. States with high malpractice rates often see migration out-of-state to other states with lower malpractice rates for specialists.

Other specialists with expensive malpractice insurance include neurosurgery and ER doctors; for others, it's not so egregious. Any physician will tell you they pay too much money for malpractice, just as many people will tell you they pay too much for car or homeowners' insurance, although many malpractice rates are actually within reason.

Primary care malpractice insurance is relatively low unless they're doing obstetrics, in part because primary care doctors don't get sued much. Again, a nuanced view from inside health care reveals the reality. Lawsuits happen when a patient has high expectations to begin with, followed by a physician's sporadic and suboptimal personal interactions with those patients and their families. Emergency room doctors who see patients once and have no real relationship with them, if they have a bad outcome with a patient, are more likely to face a lawsuit than a family doctor with an ongoing relationship of trust over the years. Primary care doctors who have established relationships with patients over years of caring for them are much more likely to be given some slack if something goes wrong. It's common sense; patients trust them, and even if they make a mistake, patients tell themselves that anyone can make a mistake. It's a completely different dynamic with a specialist, whom the patient is trusting for a dangerous, costly, once-in-a-lifetime procedure.

The malpractice issue is further complicated by contingency fees, which are against the law in other countries such as England. Barristers in England understand that it's a conflict of interest to charge based on contingency. With contingency fees, there are no out-of-pocket costs to the plaintiff, so there's no disincentive to suing. Trivial complaints end up entering litigation; and because trial lawyers make a percentage up to 35% of whatever they win, the higher the lawsuit, the better. From that standpoint, there's no question that malpractice insurance and malpractice lawsuits affect the overall cost of health care. If you watch any TV at all, you see the ads asking, "Did you take this drug? If so, you could be entitled to money, so call us at this number." Frivolous lawsuits by consumers, at times seemingly encouraged by the pharmaceutical and medical device industries, clearly exacerbate the overall cost problem.

The malpractice complexities are exacerbated by the current hospital peer-review process, which is fraught with conflicts of interest. Let's say that as a cardiologist, I have a case that goes before peer review; there's some question about whether I did the right thing or not. Who's sitting on the panel? Other cardiologists in the hospital. So either my competitors or my partners are judging me. Can either one actually be objective? There's also the collegial issue: Members of peer-review committees know that, one day, they could be under review, and the current reviewee will be sitting in judgment of them. There's a built-in incentive to be lenient when fellow doctors make mistakes, coupled with the lack of objectivity just walking into the peer review to decide whether a mistake has been made.

So the peer-review process itself is flawed but mandatory under current regulations. Issues that would be better evaluated by objective physicians end up being adjudicated in courts by contingency-incentivized malpractice lawyers. The legal system has issues that need to be reformed, but we as physicians have lacked the leadership to resolve the clinical, collegial, and practical issues with malpractice, so we're responsible for our part in the malpractice crisis.

To what degree is the malpractice issue – either the cost of insurance to physicians or the overall costs for litigation – a major factor in the healthcare crisis? While egregious medical malpractice stories make the headlines as sensational media stories, this isn't a top-tier issue in overall healthcare costs. The malpractice system needs reforming, but you could solve the malpractice dilemma tomorrow and you wouldn't solve the healthcare crisis. It's similar to "the uninsured" issue; it's a political hot-button that gets a lot of sound bites. But eliminating malpractice insurance wouldn't solve the double-digit inflation of healthcare costs because physicians still face ratcheted-down reimbursement and financial incentives to find other ways of making money within the system. We'd still have winners and losers in health care, with incentives to utilize extremely expensive technology whenever possible.

Lawyers might argue that reforming malpractice litigation would inevitably lead to even more medical errors. A broader vision might see that it may be time to rethink our contingency-based legal system. Physician leadership can play a role here in helping to reduce the unnecessary costs involved with resolving potential malpractice cases and to reduce the volume of frivolous cases seeking legal resolution.

Chapter 5
Physicians and Recent Efforts at Reform

The history of healthcare reform in our country has been long, contentious, and sharply divided, but one thing it has never been is filled with physicians at the table leading change. The future of the Affordable Care Act (ACA) of 2010 is uncertain, given the shift in Congress toward Republican politics after the 2010 midterm elections, with many Republicans vowing to repeal that reform. Because state governments would need to be centrally involved in the key structural reform in the ACA – creating the so-called "insurance exchanges" – a continued swing toward the Republican camp at the state level promises to challenge further and even erode various provisions of the recent reform – as well as propose new alternatives. To evaluate recent reform legislation and future strategies that may soon follow, it helps to understand the key issues and features of the ACA from the insiders' perspective – that of working physicians who provide care.

The fundamental issue with the lack of physician drivers in healthcare reform is that people setting policy don't have boots on the ground; they can't fully understand the nuances of clinical care. A lot of economists and policy makers have been involved in drafting healthcare reform – smart people with good ideas who can't see the clinical implications of what's now happening in medicine. Too many armchair generals and policy wonks generated proposals that ultimately killed Bill Clinton's healthcare plan, too; it wasn't driven primarily by the people practicing medicine. If the physicians on the ground don't get involved in drafting reform, then various proposals, mandates, and laws will continue to be riddled with assumptions that are just that: assumptions.

Granted, physicians haven't done a good job of transitioning to an organizational mindset and model of care, partly because there's no real economic incentive to do so. Take, for example, the effect of disruptive physician behavior. In physician groups, when a problem physician creates interpersonal difficulties for patients and staff so often that they're leaving the practice and damaging the business, there's a low threshold to taking that guy to the woodshed. The practice leader will talk to that doctor, no matter how uncomfortable the conversation is.

But when a problem physician works in a hospital, physicians don't see it as their business; they don't have to hire the replacement staff. Physicians don't own the problem and don't see any reason, except to protect themselves, to get involved. It becomes a reactive, rather than proactive, stance.

Some academic physicians, such as Arnold S. Relman, MD, the former editor-in-chief of *The New England Journal of Medicine* who has become a national healthcare policy expert, have written letters to *The New York Times,* suggesting that physicians join salaried, not-for-profit group practices and accept capitated payments. Relman views the act of physicians charging for their services in a fee-for-service model as an outright, inherent conflict of interest. He was instrumental in trying to keep pharmaceutical reps out of doctors' offices and to keep hospital pharmacy budgets from entertaining physicians, but he hasn't focused his critique on the relationship between doctors and hospitals, a relationship that has much to do with out-of-control costs.

The missing piece of healthcare reform, which well-meaning professionals outside of clinical practice often miss, is that even hospitals that employ physicians on salary, including not-for-profit organizations, still have inadequate control over physician spending. Without a bundled payment scheme, where all providers are at risk for over-wasteful behaviors, physicians can order and utilize resources that cost the system billions of dollars. Our healthcare system may ultimately end up with salaried, multispecialty, not-for-profit group practices, but the current dysfunctional fee-for-service reimbursement model has to be dismantled to control costs.

How to evaluate reform

None of the recent healthcare proposals adequately focus on the cost issue. To one degree or another, they share a lack of understanding of a key driver of overall costs: physician utilization of healthcare resources. In health care, we haven't yet clarified the cost problem, and any workable solutions will be secondary to that. Until we as a country address the cost issue, we may slip eventually into a single-party-payer system out of financial necessity. But with input and leadership from clinicians, we can do much better than defaulting to a single-party payer. Many aspects of our system and what we're doing are worth preserving, but there's a limited window of opportunity to do so.

In evaluating reform proposals from a physician's perspective, the Affordable Care Act of 2010 is not the only reform with worthwhile ideas. According to the nonpartisan Kaiser Family Foundation's analysis of major reform proposals in recent years, a different plan, led by bipartisan Senate majority leaders Howard Baker, Tom Daschle, and Bob Dole, suggested a move away from the fee-for-service model in our country. The Baker-Daschle-Dole plan is the only recent proposal to suggest dropping the fee-for-service model and expanding the use of bundled payments beyond Medicare and Medicaid to physicians. Eliminating fee-for-service is the only mechanism that will control costs enough to make a difference in the national budget.

Because it focuses on accessibility rather than cost, the Affordable Care Act (ACA) doesn't adequately address overall national healthcare costs. When the Kaiser Family Foundation recently did a survey on Americans' understanding of the new plan and what they most liked about it, "easy-to-understand plan summaries" from insurers came out on top. Clearly, the cost implications of the Affordable Care Act aren't uppermost in Americans' minds, although in 2011 insurance premiums for U.S. families rose by 9%, up from the typical 5% annual rate increase. While the Kaiser Family Foundation attributes only 1% to 2% of the increase to the ACA, specifically to the provisions that allow parents' policies to cover children through age 26 and that require certain policies to provide preventive care at no cost, the ability of the ACA to solve the overall cost issue is questionable at best.

There's an opportunity and responsibility here as citizens – not to be partisan and criticize a given Democratic or Republican solution – but rather to look objectively at the cost implications of various reform ideas. Many Americans find themselves on a steep learning curve when it comes to educating themselves about how health care really works, now that costs have spiraled so far out of control that they're impossible to ignore. Consumers, physicians, and hospital executives are all scratching their heads trying to digest and evaluate the fiscal implications of the Affordable Care Act, along with critical provisions being challenged and possibly overridden in future political climates. Many of the ACA reforms aren't scheduled to go into effect until 2014 or later, so the time is ripe to clarify and modify any provisions in healthcare reform that don't resolve the national cost issue.

The driving concern is cost – and motivating people to think and talk about cost – that's the lens through which I evaluate reform plans. But my experience in discussing healthcare reform with physicians, hospital leadership, and politicians has proven what a hot issue it has become. Supporters of the ACA reform became so vested in it that they promoted it as an unequivocal, major victory. It may be seen as a victory to increase access to care, but it fails to address long-term healthcare costs adequately. In fact, the ACA increases the regulatory burden and therefore the bureaucratic expenses of health care. It relies heavily on centralized decision-making regarding outcomes and does not enable providers the practical creativity needed to define clinical value.

Depending on the political process rather than providers to define a solution has further complicated the situation. Discussing the Affordable Care Act has become polarizing, almost a litmus test some people use to judge whether you're a fair-minded progressive or a narrow-minded reactionary. Until there's more agreement on what the problem is – understanding the real drivers of cost and the unnecessary utilization of expensive technology, coupled with workable financial incentives for behavioral change and effective leadership development among physicians – the likely default "solution" cannot adequately resolve the current crisis.

Assumptions in healthcare reform

Access and cost.

The biggest flaw from a physician's perspective in the Affordable Care Act is the assumption that giving healthcare access to more individuals will reduce overall costs. This assumes that because people would have insurance and could go to a primary care doctor sooner, they could reduce costly emergency room visits and avoid catastrophic illness. But there's no data to suggest that this is true. In fact, in February 2012, the Associated Press/*Businessweek* reported that in the federal budget for fiscal year 2013, Medicare spending would double over the next 10 years from $478 billion to nearly $1 *trillion* in 2022. During the same period, Medicaid would more than double, from $255 billion to $589 billion by 2022.

Consumers who aren't accessing health care right now obviously spend little or nothing on medical care, so they're living with bad hips, chronic pain, untreated diabetes, unrepaired hernias, cataracts, and a host of other chronic conditions. Suspending ethical perspectives for a moment to focus on cost, the reality is that these "untreated patients" aren't included in current spending on health care as a percentage of

GDP. If you give millions of people new access to health care and they use it, assuming that the currently insured will continue to utilize care at the same or greater capacity, it can only drive up costs. By how much? We don't yet know, but it likely will be considerable given what happened in Massachusetts when inappropriate utilization of emergency rooms continued despite increased coverage, and overall healthcare costs rose. That state is now considering other cost-containment measures, such as a proposal to do away with fee-for-service reimbursement.

So there's precedence that increasing access to health care increases overall costs, not only from the Massachusetts example but also from our country's history of access and costs. Back in the 1950s when no one had insurance, health care made up 1% of GDP. With the advent of private insurance and government-sponsored health care through Medicare, utilization and spending rose exponentially. Covering millions more Americans will likely lead to the same outcome.

Prevention and cost.

A second shaky assumption is that spending more money on prevention will reduce healthcare costs. In fact, there are few diseases with high-quality, consistent data proving that prevention reduces cost. Vaccinating children is one of the few preventive measures that has consistently positive outcomes: Once you vaccinate children for rubella, for instance, they're not going to get rubella. But few prevention measures are as cut-and-dried or as proven as vaccination.

The overwhelming majority of clinical studies on prevention have researched "secondary" prevention – prevention protocols with patients who already have a disease. We don't have much good data on the medical implications of treating people who are "at risk" but don't yet have disease. "Primary" prevention (prevention efforts before disease manifests) in the general population might work; it might not. Money spent in prevention might be a good investment or not; we don't yet know.

Even in the few areas where science does eventually prove that prevention works and does reduce costs, the next rational question must be *when* it will reduce costs. Any prevention data usually suggests a cost reduction over the long term, but the healthcare crisis is more urgent. While it's clearly of clinical benefit if prevention saves money 30 years from now, our healthcare system won't survive that long to find out. Exploding costs have to be addressed immediately, not 30 years from now. There's not enough quality data on prevention to bank on its actually having a major impact on cost, and we can't compete globally if we continue to spend nearly 18% of GDP on health care – and rising. The Centers for Medicare and Medicaid estimate healthcare spending to rise to 19.6% of GDP in 2019.

Insurance reforms and cost.

The third faulty assumption is that setting up competition between two radically different entities – private insurers on the one hand and a government insurance option on the other –would lower private insurance costs. The Affordable Care Act limits how much money private insurers can put into their investment pools as financial reserves, but a safe level of reserves is what makes the insurance industry viable. Private insurers with government-imposed limits on reserves cannot compete with federal plans that have essentially unlimited reserves through the government's ability to raise revenues by increasing taxes or by printing more money. It's an uneven playing field.

Of more concern, because the proposed penalty to employers for not providing health care under the Affordable Care Act is less expensive than the price of most healthcare policies, the ACA incentivizes employers not to provide insurance, which would likely push more consumers into the new government plans. The government has proven it has little ability to control healthcare costs; as healthcare analysts continue to point out, Medicare and Medicaid, the "single-party-payer systems" we now have, are already in crisis. It doesn't make sense to add millions of people into a system that's already mismanaged and in financial crisis as a cost-containment strategy.

"Fraud and abuse" and cost.

A fourth faulty assumption is that we can keep Medicare afloat by eliminating millions of dollars of fraud and abuse. As discussed earlier, there's not enough real fraud and abuse in the system to pay the enormous growth in funding needed to expand Medicare and Medicaid. A better focus for Medicare savings would be to evaluate the waste that Medicare pays for by using the old fee-for-service system that incentivizes for overutilization.

Reform ideas: a single-party payer

Growing a larger federal and state healthcare system raises the ongoing debate about the pros and cons of moving toward a single-party-payer system. Arnold Relman, MD, formerly of *The New England Journal of Medicine*, has expressed a commonly shared concern about the possibility of a single-party-payer system in a letter to *The New York Times*, arguing that our experience with Medicare proves that a single-party-payer structure doesn't work to control costs. Other physicians have written to the *Times* and countless other periodicals supporting a single-party payer. That various types of physicians – primary care, specialty care, academic physicians – view a single-payer system differently should come as no surprise given that the current financial incentive system has created winners and losers in the physician community.

I sit on the Executive Committee for the King County Medical Society with other physicians, most of whom who are in practice, with a proportionately small number of academic physicians. We debate proposals to put into the plank for the Washington State Medical Association, and at a recent meeting one doctor brought up the idea of supporting a single-party payer, which didn't go far. He was a primary care physician, and a single-party payer makes sense for him, but the specialists in the group were livid over that possibility.

In physicians' minds, the one benefit of a single-party payer would be to reduce the paperwork of current medical regulations, which have grown significantly enough to cost physicians time and overhead in their practices. Physicians have never been fans of putting bureaucrats in charge of making medical decisions; but the growth of the regulatory environment has grown beyond merely off-putting to unwieldy, time-consuming, and a negative hit on their bottom lines.

Prospective, capitated payments to integrated healthcare systems would address both spiraling costs and out-of-control bureaucratic regulations. By rewarding providers for delivering cost-effective care with bundled, lump-sum payments and keeping bureaucrats out of the mix, providers would figure out how to make the finances work. Ultimately, a single-party-payer system may be where we're heading due to the growing crisis in the provider community and the systemic fatigue from constant financial uncertainty. The current lack of physician leadership in shaping the debate and building consensus to create real solutions all but guarantee a single-party payer as the only remaining option – but we can, and should, do better.

Reform ideas: bundled payments

CMS (the Centers for Medicare & Medicaid) has started a pilot bundled-payment initiative, which links payments for multiple services that patients receive during a single episode of care. Instead of a procedure generating multiple claims from multiple providers, the entire team is compensated with a bundled payment that provides incentives to deliver healthcare services more efficiently while maintaining or improving quality of care. Participation in the pilot program is voluntary. Since it's likely that the program will result in significant savings to CMS, it could quickly become the standard for reimbursement for all CMS services, in the absence of a national rush toward other reform initiatives such as the formation of Accountable Care Organizations (ACOs).

The adoption of either initiative as a standard – bundled payments for episodes of care or widespread ACOs – would effectively abolish the current fee-for-service method of payment for physician payments and do away with the current division between Medicare Part A and Part B reimbursement. Both solutions would require a level of healthcare integration on the part of providers that is, thus far, extremely rare in the current environment. Physician leaders will be challenged to create, manage, and maintain models of care that distribute responsibilities and resources in a manner that creates value – quality divided by cost – requiring new levels of collaborative behavior unprecedented in health care to date.

Reform ideas: universal coverage

President Barack Obama, passionate about the nearly 50 million uninsured people in the United States, centered his initial healthcare reform debate on that injustice. The uninsured is a form of social injustice that the country can't minimize and needs to address, but covering the uninsured wouldn't solve the healthcare crisis, which has to address overall cost.

In the 2008 presidential campaign, Barack Obama and Hillary Clinton both argued to cover all Americans with health insurance. Clinton argued that it should be mandatory; Obama argued that it should be optional. The difference between those two positions is relatively small politically, but it does go to the issue of cost and how health care would be paid for. The idea of providing all Americans with health care began with Teddy Roosevelt and continued with Presidents Truman and Nixon; they believed that just as no one should be starving in America, no one should have to go without health care.

That's the ideal. The reality is that we're spending too much of our GDP on health care, and health care costs are outpacing inflation by an exponential amount – a cost we can't afford to sustain. Adding people to the insurance pool before solving the cost problem can only exacerbate the fiscal crisis.

Going into the 2008 presidential election, the Democrats identified *a* problem, but they didn't identify *the* problem: They didn't focus on escalating costs. On the Republican side, Tim Pawlenty (R-MN), who briefly ran for president in the spring of 2011, was interviewed after one of Obama's speeches supporting healthcare reform, and Pawlenty challenged his healthcare focus, arguing that the real issue was cost. Few reporters picked up on that story at the time. But when that challenge came back to the Democratic Party and to then-Senator Obama, they began claiming that by offering insurance to everyone, they'd reduce healthcare costs; Obama said this several times during his initial presidential campaign. It's one of those sound bites that sounds as if it could be true, but in fact – without first addressing overall costs – is not.

Supporters of universal coverage often argue that when you offer insurance to the uninsured, they'll stop overutilizing expensive resources such as emergency rooms; they'll seek care earlier with less inappropriate utilization of catastrophic and emergency care, the most expensive kinds of care. That all sounds logical in a sound bite – except that there's no data to support the claim.

In fact, many people who show up at emergency departments with trivial complaints do have insurance. They come to the ED for other reasons, often for convenience so they don't miss work or will be seen more quickly than waiting for a primary care appointment. On the other hand, a lot of uninsured Americans have multiple, chronic medical conditions that they're not receiving care for, so while that's a societal and ethical issue, from a systemic cost perspective, they're also not spending healthcare dollars. For the nearly 50 million Americans who don't have insurance, a significant number of which have serious untreated medical issues, as soon as they have affordable insurance they're likely to seek medical care to treat those conditions. If we don't address the cost issue as our first priority, increasing the availability of insurance can only raise overall healthcare costs.

Democratic plans have called for "taxing the rich" to pay for reform, although it's unclear whose revenue numbers make sense, since it's impossible to predict the ongoing national cost of insuring 50 million uninsured Americans. On the other hand, it's hard to be enthusiastic about the solution from Republicans. Senator John McCain (R-AZ), the Republican presidential nominee in the 2008 election, proposed to reduce healthcare costs by letting consumers spend their own money. Republicans spearheaded the idea of pretax Health Savings Accounts, along with tax credits, to let consumers buy their own health insurance and figure out for themselves how to spend that money. As discussed previously, this kind of argument treats health care as a commodity; our society does not. Furthermore, given the actual dollars needed to pay out-of-pocket for an angioplasty at $38,000, for example, the average person likely wouldn't have that much cash on hand to spend, just by putting away a few thousand dollars into a Health Savings Account over the years.

Reform ideas: prevention to control costs

Reform pundits play on misconceptions in consumers' minds when they state unequivocally that more prevention services will reduce healthcare expenses. It sounds reasonable to the uninitiated, but there's little data to support that claim. It *may*. But preventive measures could increase overall costs, as well.

It's unclear in the final analysis, for example, whether more frequent mammograms actually reduce morbidity and mortality due to breast cancer, which is why the recommendations for mammography keep changing. For decades physicians thought that all middle-aged men needed a PSA (prostate-specific antigen) test to screen for prostate cancer. Now researchers are finding that they don't know what to do with the test data; there doesn't seem to be a clear relationship between death rates and PSA results. Many researchers now recommend less frequent PSA tests since it's unclear how picking up a prostate cancer early actually benefits patients, given that the cure can be worse than the disease.

The explosion in the use of diagnostic imaging comes into play here. The latest technologies such as 3D mammography have become increasingly sensitive, so for the average consumer it's logical to think that medicine can now detect smaller cancers earlier and assume that's a good thing. But more sensitive imaging systems also generate more "false positive" test results, so more unnecessary procedures, such as lumpectomies of the breast, are performed.

CT scans from head to toe can detect all sorts of "abnormalities" early on – and for a while some providers were advocating this – but the question becomes what useful action anyone could take with that information. It's not clear. In medicine, most studies have been done on disease; it's less clear what happens with healthy, asymptomatic people and "pre-disease." From the clinicians' standpoint, then, we look at the argument that more prevention will automatically save money for the overall system and know that's not necessarily true.

Reform ideas: market competition

One of the reform ideas continually bantered about is market competition: Let the market fairly decide who's a winner and loser in health care. But because health care is not a commodity, allowing healthcare plans to compete may not actually lower costs; the market competition model may not hold up in health care. In the manufacturing sector, to compete and make more sofas and sell them for less, you could use cheaper material, lower the quality, price your product lower, or use less labor to save money. The consumer would be faced with a value proposition: buy a top-end sofa of better material at one store and spend 20 times more money, go somewhere else and spend less on something that's not top-end but workable, or not buy a sofa at all and sit on the floor.

That "commodity thinking" doesn't work in health care. Healthcare plans, hospitals, and doctors can't provide truly substandard service. There's a certain baseline quality that medical providers have to maintain. So we're trending toward what's happening with the airlines, where the quality of the experience plummets. The airlines aren't crashing more now that they're competing; they're still safe, but the consumer experience of flying has changed considerably for the worse, along with additional costs passed on to consumers, literally from soup to nuts.

In many ways, this is happening in health care. If we don't change the way doctors are reimbursed and instead squeeze tighter on how much money doctors are paid per patient or per procedure, physicians' response will be to increase throughput. That's the rational response, and it's the reason doctors now have so little time to spend with patients. Because physicians are incredibly stressed by the reimbursement squeeze – every minute counts – they've had to schedule patient visits at increasingly shorter and shorter intervals.

The market competition model that works for other industries can't simply be transplanted onto health care under the current reimbursement system. Health care is a unique market for multiple reasons, not the least of which is that providers don't have the option to offer a marginal, inferior product, or no product at all. The ethical, professional, and legal issues in medicine are truly unique. If we as a society ratchet down overall spending and force physicians and hospitals to reevaluate how they're providing care – in effect, forcing them to create a better value proposition – that's one thing. But because the system has ratcheted down physician reimbursement across the board, without changing the fee-for-service system, it has pushed physicians and hospitals to look for services that produce more profitable, high-tech procedures, and to bypass or minimize services that produce less profit through direct patient care.

Key features of recent reform

Accountable Care Organizations (ACOs).

Two federal initiatives in the Patient Protection and Affordable Care Act signed into law in 2010 will likely change the current financial incentives in health care soon: Accountable Care Organizations and Medicare bundled payments. The sound financial logic of both of these initiatives is likely to survive regardless of the long-term fate of the overall bill.

Section 3022 of the Affordable Care Act requires the Centers for Medicare & Medicaid Services (CMS) to establish financial incentives to integrate care through a shared savings program. The program is voluntary, offering potentially better Medicare reimbursement for providers. In order to participate, eligible providers, hospitals, and suppliers would have to come together and create Accountable Care

Organizations (ACOs), which lie at the heart of the structural reforms in the Affordable Care Act. ACOs align the financial incentives of all their members, putting all participants at risk for poor outcomes and rewarding all for outcome improvements. While the current financial incentives don't appear to many current healthcare organizations to justify the investment needed to fulfill the ACO requirements, this will no doubt change as CMS continues to reduce payments to those who choose not to participate. But Accountable Care Organizations may ultimately become another example of trying to fix health care with more layers of bureaucrats, in which both doctors and hospitals have to report their "performance" and bureaucrats evaluate those results to decide whether or not to pay for that care.

Roughly 15 years ago, some of the private insurance companies – and for a brief time, even Medicare – attempted to put a cap on healthcare costs through "capitated" care, a form of managed care. It fell apart; it became a PR nightmare. One woman was sent home from the hospital, for instance, too soon after delivering her baby and had major medical issues, and the media reported that the healthcare system was withholding proper care to make money. "Capitation" basically disappeared as a healthcare policy term; but it's coming back, dressed up as a new concept: Accountable Care Organizations. While ACOs play centerstage in recent healthcare legislation, it's worth noting that a significant number of healthcare providers don't believe ACOs will succeed due to the high "cost to play" in meeting unrealistic organizational, operational, and reporting expectations. Needless to say, those expectations were set not by physician and hospital leaders, but by policy makers.

To be certified as an Accountable Care Organization, an integrated system made up of a network of physicians tied to a hospital would have to meet a range of operational, administrative, and clinical criteria, with revamped systems, such as electronic medical records, up and running quickly. These new ACO entities must also include a legal means to account for and distribute any shared savings they may generate by providing efficient care.

Clinicians are rightly concerned about one of the key ideas behind ACOs: measuring "performance." The ACO would report its performance based on measures designated by the government, and based on those results, the ACO's payment would go up or down – a worthwhile intention, but perhaps unrealistic without enough familiarity with clinical realities. Clinical outcomes research is a fledgling science. Clinical medicine still has a long way to go, in practice, before medical knowledge is fully verified with strong outcomes data and consistently disseminated down through physicians' ranks. Along with the issue of variables in physician prescribing and treating behavior, clinical outcomes data also depends on huge "*x* factors" on the part of patients, such as medical history, compliance with prescribed treatment, contributing lifestyle factors, and other uncontrollable variables in patients' behavior.

Among the members of our region's Congressional District Health Care Advisory Board, none of the biggest healthcare systems in our area, at the time of this writing, plans to invest in becoming an ACO. Further, no ACO bureaucracy exists right now, so the government would need to fund and develop a new bureaucracy from the ground up. Where would that money come from? Health care is already a highly complicated system, and it's further complicated by inviting more bureaucrats to the table, rather than training physicians to be leaders in creating a new, sustainable system.

The professionals who provide clinical care are the people with the best training, expertise, and clinical know-how to figure out how to make the best parts of our system work without bankrupting the country. But when physicians look at the current reform law that was passed in 2010 and how it plans to contain costs, many of them see nothing but more bureaucracy so complicated that it can't possibly work to control overall spending. The idea of Accountable Care Organizations may fall apart because even those providers who want to do it can't; they see the mandates and timelines as unreasonable. When I chaired the fall 2011 meeting of the Eighth Congressional District Healthcare Advisory Committee, the physicians and regional hospital leaders agreed that it's an unworkable provision as written, and at that time, none of the represented provider systems in King County were moving ahead to do it.

As the summary of the law states, "To qualify as an ACO, organizations must agree to be accountable for the overall care of their Medicare beneficiaries, have adequate participation of primary care physicians, define processes to promote evidence-based medicine, report on quality and costs, and coordinate care." The joke for physicians and hospitals is that the incentive to satisfy all that bureaucracy and administration is so low, it's nonexistent: The "incentive" offered is to allow the ACO to "share in the cost savings they achieve for the Medicare program." Clinicians know that in the current system, sharing in the "savings" from taking care of Medicare patients is a losing proposition.

It's easy for politicians sitting at 30,000 feet to require a change such as electronic medical records to improve health information technology. As an idea, it makes good sense. The reality: Federal regulations such as the Health Insurance Portability and Accountability Act of 1996 (HIPAA) set forth privacy and security rules that make health information technology hugely complicated, on top of an already chaotic healthcare information technology environment. It would take years to remodel, reprogram, and link the technology the way it could work – and the way the ACA legislation mandates that it work.

When I was Chief Medical Officer at the Lumedx Corporation, a leading cardiovascular systems software company, I went with colleagues to some of the most prestigious hospitals around the country to promote our information technology product for their cardiology reporting systems. At one of the most highly respected research hospitals in the nation, the cardiology department alone had nearly 110 proprietary databases – none of which communicated with each other – and the overwhelming majority of which weren't even secure. They had doctors walking out of the hospital with data on their laptops that could have put them in violation of HIPAA regulations. Just to coax that one department to agree on an information technology language that could communicate among systems was a lengthy, Herculean task.

Within most hospitals, there are hundreds of databases that aren't linked to each other, but politicians toss around the idea of simply going to the Internet, linking in, and showing everyone everywhere what they need to see. While it's imperative that healthcare systems move toward much greater data sharing, the government's mandate that it be done by a specific date is unworkable – and providers recognize that. When my colleagues in King County, Washington, initially looked at the reform plan, they considered becoming an ACO; but when they evaluated their own operational systems and what it would take to participate, they realized they couldn't possibly meet the deadlines in the mandate. If the largest, most successful healthcare systems in the Seattle region can't afford to become an ACO, what will happen in smaller, less medically sophisticated communities?

Though the American Recovery and Reinvestment Act of 2009 had already made electronic medical records a national priority, in reality there's been a stand-off between the ACO idea and hospitals who can't meet the new mandate as written. The government claims it will penalize hospitals for not meeting the mandate, but many hospital leaders have figured out that the penalty will cost them less than compliance. A study of electronic medical records published in *The New England Journal of Medicine* in 2009 reported that only 1.5% of U.S. hospitals at that time had a comprehensive electronic records system in all clinical units, and another 7.6% had a "basic" system, meaning in at least one clinical unit. That same study found that only 17% of hospitals had implemented computerized physician order entry (CPOE) for medications across all clinical units. A key barrier to adoption, hospitals reported, was physician resistance. Getting physicians to use a hospital-based computerized system proves a huge task – and it's key to the success of ACOs.

American Health Benefit Exchanges.

The Affordable Care Act calls for creating government-run healthcare plans called American Health Benefit Exchanges to compete with private insurers, with government-subsidized risk pools for low-income people at 133% to 400% of federal poverty level. (The plan assumes that people below that income level will already be on Medicaid or at least have access to it.) These state-run insurance Exchanges would funnel federal funding to states, which are then charged with creating and operating the Exchanges. Individuals and small businesses would buy coverage through these Exchanges.

The net effect clearly would be a much larger government-run system of health care, federally subsidized as Medicare is now subsidized but operated by the states. It's unclear from the plan how past operational and financial management issues with Medicare and Medicaid will be circumvented with the Exchanges. In fact, the ACA builds on the state-run Medicaid model, with federal funds paying for the increased numbers of people who qualify for Medicaid coverage. The new law essentially requires states to cover nearly all of its low-income residents under age 65 and pay into risk pools for the individual and small business markets. The Congressional Budget Office has estimated that the ACA would ultimately extend coverage to about 32 million people, roughly half through Medicaid expansion and half through the expansion of private insurance.

A December 2010 analysis by the nonpartisan, research-based Urban Institute estimated that the ACA will raise state budgets between about $21 billion and $43 billion between 2014 and 2019, but that given potential savings in the reform plan (such as shifting Medicaid adults to the Exchanges), the net effect could save state budgets between $41 billion and $132 billion during those same years. But again, from a physician's perspective, the faulty assumptions behind access, prevention, fraud and abuse, and other reform ideas make those numbers suspect.

Expanding Medicaid.

At the same time, however, the Affordable Care Act also calls for expanding Medicaid to 133% of federal poverty level, which would radically increase the number of people on Medicaid. The potential of reducing state expenditures by a plan that could move people from Medicaid to the new federal insurance Exchanges is of little comfort to state governors and legislators, already forced to deal with an immediate increase in expenditures given the mandate that moves more people into Medicaid.

A state-funded initiative, Medicaid has been disastrously unaffordable to most state governments for years. At the passage of the ACA, many state governors rebelled and sued the federal government over the Medicaid provision, concerned about extending a program that has long operated in the red. Unlike the federal government with Medicare, states have to balance their budgets; they can't balance their budgets by adding millions of people to their healthcare spending, and they can't go into deficit spending to cover a Medicaid expansion. Again, it illustrates the distortion of media sound bites, which showed politicians slapping each other on the back and saying, "We expanded healthcare access for all." But they failed to explain how, at what cost – and with whose wallet.

When Republicans rose to power in Congress in 2011, they began submitting their own counterproposals to challenge healthcare reform and fight Medicare expansion. The budget proposal by Representative Paul Ryan, adopted by the House in April 2011, focused on cutting federal spending for health care by turning Medicaid into a block grant to states and limiting any increase in Medicaid funding paid to states based on population growth and the consumer price index, rather than on actual healthcare costs or expanding coverage. Time will tell how future challenges to the ACA will play out on Capitol Hill.

The Affordable Care Act also requires states to increase their Medicaid reimbursement to primary care physicians, but states can't afford the reimbursement they're now paying. According to Pulitzer Prize-winning author and sociologist Paul Starr writing in *Remedy and Reaction: The Peculiar American Struggle over Health Care Reform*, Medicaid costs the states about 20% less than private insurance does, so it's hard to imagine finding savings or keeping Medicaid afloat without an infusion of funding. Medicare payment rates to doctors and hospitals are just as dismal, typically running at 20% to 30% of private insurance rates.

The reality in medicine today: Financing the expanded coverage of Medicaid through decreasing federal payments to the states every year is a problematic model. The federal government is slated to pay "100%" of this provision for 2014 through 2016, but it's increasing the states' requirement beyond "100%," since states would have two new responsibilities: to increase the number of people who qualify for Medicaid and to pay more for physicians' services. In essence, then, this provision would doubly increase the total healthcare costs for states.

As states already struggle to make Medicaid work, they're paying Medicaid rates so low that most physicians can't afford to accept them. What Medicaid currently reimburses physicians ends up being a loss, so even if doctors can take on a few Medicaid patients out of beneficence, they have to limit their Medicaid patients to a minute percentage of billings. While the ACA does suggest a small increase in fees to primary care doctors, those physicians still will be seeing patients "below cost" in a money-losing proposition that's unsustainable to many of them. Without changing the current fee-for-structure paradigm and incentivizing toward value, these minor fixes are more bandaids on a hemorrhage.

With these low Medicaid payments to physicians, many states already have trouble keeping their Medicaid programs afloat. Given the current economy, with more people living at or near the poverty level, Medicaid ranks are likely to swell. What kind of leverage is Medicaid going to have in the marketplace when it's expanded, given the current, unworkable, even contentious relationship with doctors? How can we ask already financially challenged primary care doctors to accept more patients to care for, below their actual costs?

The ACA also calls for expansion of other public healthcare programs, such as the Children's Health Insurance Program (CHIP), a federally funded program that helps provide basic health care for children by cost sharing with states. In the ACA, what looks at first glance to be an improvement – a 23% increase in CHIP payments – has a cap at 100%. Since CHIP reimbursement is already at a 50% discount, in reality it only raises reimbursement to where it should have been all along.

"The uninsured" has become such a political hot button, though, that anyone suggesting that our country can't afford to insure all of the uninsured gets tarred and feathered. Few people really know what health care actually costs and how the money's changing hands, which is why "insuring the uninsured" is the wrong focus. Expanding care is inarguably a noble idea, but it's not addressing the problem: We can't afford the system as it stands now. Without a clear vision of quality and value, we can't make the tough systemic choices that will give us the most bang for our collective healthcare buck in the long term.

The individual mandate.

One of the most contentious provisions of healthcare reform is the "individual mandate," which requires nearly all U.S. citizens to have health insurance or to pay an annual tax penalty. As of this writing, the individual mandate has been challenged as unconstitutional; three federal judges have upheld it, two have struck it down. The ACA would phase in the penalty to consumers beginning with $95 in 2014 and rising to $695 in 2016, to a maximum of $2,085 per family (or assessed according to a percentage of taxable income).

To avoid paying the penalty, people living at 133% to 400% of federal poverty level could buy into the proposed American Health Benefit Exchange plans, which would be kept at low cost and subsidized by the government. But exemptions to the individual mandate, broadly defined, include financial hardship. People already near the poverty level, who can't afford the relatively low cost of buying into the government-sponsored insurance plan each year, may choose to pay the $695 penalty because it's the lower amount; so the ACA essentially incentivizes them to continue going to the ER for expensive care even when their medical condition isn't acute. Another financial sinkhole would stem from the administrative costs of trying to collect those penalties from people living near the poverty level who can't afford them.

Other stated exemptions to the individual mandate include American Indians and undocumented immigrants, who don't have to buy insurance but can still use hospital emergency rooms, since hospitals bear an ethical obligation to provide emergency care to whomever comes through the door. Ultimately, the reform legislation, like many political solutions required to get a bill passed, is full of exceptions and loopholes; it's an open checkbook.

Disincentives for employer coverage.

While the Affordable Care Act ostensibly requires employers with 50 or more fulltime employees to offer coverage, in reality, it effectively incentivizes companies not to hire fulltime employees, because companies would have to pay a penalty of $2,000 for every fulltime employee they don't cover with insurance (excluding the first 30 employees).

What would happen to companies spending more than $2,000 on health insurance per employee? They may either fire their fulltime employees or pay the penalty instead of providing medical benefits, because the penalty would cost them less than providing insurance. Company CEOs who don't currently cover their employees may know that it's not the right thing to do; but with the ACA, if a company pays the penalty, those employees now qualify for the government plan because they don't have insurance – so the CEO's decision may look a little less morally egregious. The private insurers won't be able to compete given the likely influx of enrollees into the federal Exchanges and the indirect incentives for funneling people into the government-run plans. But spin doctors sold the ACA by promising that it would in no way affect insurance for people already satisfied with their plans – a misleading sound bite for the public.

Premium subsidies.

Not only does the Affordable Care Act call for government-sponsored insurance plans, it also offers subsidies to consumers to buy them.

The ACA would increase these premium cost-sharing subsidies over time based on premium increases, so the government won't be able to control premium-cost growth – clearly driving up federal spending on health care over time.

The plan also gives tax credits to employers, including small companies with relatively small wages, to help them afford insurance for their employees. But as discussed, it will cost employers more to offer insurance than pay the penalty, which is only $2,000 per employee – a penalty much lower than the typical annual cost to cover an employee.

Tax changes to private insurance.

The ACA carries a tax penalty on insurers for their high-end, "Cadillac" insurance plans, a tax that will in turn affect consumers and their rates. This provision calls for insurers to pay an excise tax to the federal government for employer-sponsored health plans with aggregate values of more than $10,200 for individual coverage or $27,500 for family coverage, effective beginning in 2018. These so-called "Cadillac" plans are actually "Chevrolet" plans, given those dollar amounts, since most large, national employers offer plans that fit this criteria.

The excise tax would be 40% of the amount of the plan that exceeds those dollar amounts, whether the insurer is a health insurance company or a large, self-insured employer. Republicans have argued that this provision would kill business, and it might; it would clearly be a huge hit for companies who have done the right thing by their employees and offered good coverage.

The ACA also calls for an increase in taxes coming out of Health Savings Accounts (HSAs), which were initially created so that consumers could spend their own pretax dollars on health care. Less incentive for individuals to put money away for medical care creates another push toward a government-run system.

Today you can use an HSA card to pay for over-the-counter medications as well as prescription drugs. The Affordable Care Act excludes using your HSA to pay for over-the-counter medications not prescribed by a doctor, which might sound like a good idea. But that provides an incentive for people who don't actually need to see a doctor to see a doctor, and who don't actually need a prescription to get a prescription. Shouldn't we incentivize people to buy their own Tylenol and Sudafed, rather than go to a doctor to save money on these products? In the new plan, people can only use an HSA card to pay for Tylenol if they go to a doctor and get a prescription for it, so it's providing incentives for unnecessary doctors' visits that the healthcare system ultimately pays for.

The Affordable Care Act increases the hospital insurance tax rate, raising the taxes hospitals have to pay, and imposes new taxes on the pharmaceutical industry, a sector that typically responds to overhead increases by passing them on to consumers. The plan also increases the insurance sector fee, which gets passed on to businesses that buy their insurance products. It's going to cost employers more if insurers have to pay more to the government to be in business. It's clearly not a level playing field for private insurers who have to pay the government – their competition – fees to compete. It's another incentive to drive consumers to the less-expensive government plan, which doesn't have those additional fees to absorb into their business costs.

In many ways, the Affordable Care Act adds layers of complexity and bureaucracy rather than simplifying the system to offer better health care at a better cost – creating higher value. But while the plan has passed into law, provisions that require funding have not yet been enabled or funded, and many aren't slated to begin until 2014 or later. The federal budget has been held in continuing resolutions to fund only existing programs, so the healthcare crisis is still very much alive. So while the ACA appropriated billions of dollars to create small-business insurance co-ops, for instance, there may never be co-ops, given the changing political climate and continued challenges to reform. Even the mandates passed into law – to expand Medicaid and to require all individuals to have health insurance via the individual mandate – are being challenged fiercely.

Other cost-containment mandates.

The ACA also calls for establishing an Independent Payment Advisory Board of 15 members to recommend ways to reduce the growth rate of Medicare spending, but the Board appears prohibited from having any power. The ACA states: "The Board is prohibited from submitting proposals that would ration care, increase revenues or change benefits, eligibility or Medicare beneficiary cost sharing (including Parts A and B premiums)," which doesn't leave the Board any room to affect changes to control costs. Further, the plan states that, "Hospitals and hospices (through 2019) and clinical labs (for one year) will not be subject to cost reductions proposed by the Board." Without any cost reductions from 2012 to 2019 in the most expensive arena of health care – hospitalizations – how will this new Board succeed in cost containment, and how will the system stay afloat? Of note, this provision requires that one member of the Board be a physician, but having only one in 15 decision-makers as a clinical professional experienced in delivering care won't make for a balanced, successful Payment Advisory Board.

Sound bite: "euthanasia for seniors"

The healthcare crisis has long been rife with misleading sound bites that cloud the debate and perpetuate the fears that drive physicians and consumers. When the Republicans slammed the ACA reform proposal, they claimed that it funded "death squads," which were supposedly groups of doctors paid to keep the elderly from accessing treatment. The "death squad" sound bite grossly misrepresented a clause in the ACA suggesting that when a physician sits and counsels patients about end-of-life issues, that doctor could bill for that time with a reimbursable patient-care code. Paying doctors to explain end-of-life care is not exactly a "death squad."

In fact, the ACA simply suggested paying physicians to do what they were already doing gratis. So instead of physicians having to rush through a two-minute conversation about the intimate, complicated issues of end-of-life care, they could sit with a patient and family, answer their questions, and be reimbursed for their time. The point of the legislation was not to encourage any one pathway through end-of-life care, but to pay the doctor – often a primary care doctor – fairly for their time.

One negative ad online purported to show "euthanasia camps" using video of President Obama responding to the idea of "death camps" for seniors, manipulated to make it appear as if he were supporting the idea. In another, actors wearing white robes were being marched by men in uniforms to a guillotine. Other ads run in the mainstream media, targeting seniors who were confused about the reform legislation, claimed that the bill was trying to "get rid of seniors" to save money. As people get older, they fear abandonment, isolation, and marginalization from society, so this sound bite played into that fear and resonated with seniors. Counseling patients on end-of-life issues, from the physicians' perspective, is part of our ethical responsibility in caring for patients, but end-of-life decisions are made – by law – by individual patients. If consumers don't know the law, they won't know that the idea of a "death panel" is illegal.

In fact, too many patients, by default, use medical resources toward the end of their lives that they don't truly want or need because they don't understand their options. From 1992 to 1996, mean annual medical expenditures during the last year of life for people aged 65 and older were five times the annual costs incurred in their nonterminal years ($37,581 versus $7,365), and last-year-of-life expenses constituted 26% of overall Medicare spending. Patients and their families might make the same treatment choices if they knew all the options, or they might not. The point is that patients have the right to know what to expect clinically at the end of their lives and to choose the medical care that matches their values.

My anecdotal evidence from my own and colleagues' clinical experience is that when you have candid conversations with people at the end of their lives and explain what's going to happen if they choose one treatment option over another – one of which may extend their lives but with extremely difficult side effects – they may choose not to do it. A 90-year-old with terminal cancer may decide that chemotherapy that brings on constant nausea, vomiting, and extreme weakness to gain an additional six months to live may not be worthwhile. Since it's the patients' choice, they deserve to know the consequences of treatment in terms of their quality of life. Elderly patients often choose not to pursue further treatment. They'll choose a better quality of life in the short term so they can enjoy that time left with their families; they don't want to be in a hospital. But the sound bites focused on "denying care" and "shipping Granny off to die." Many physicians, ironically, found that being reimbursed for counseling patients on end-of-life care was one of the few things in the ACA they could all agree with.

It's a public responsibility to see through politically motivated sound bites that distort the realities of healthcare policy. Is there value in doctors counseling patients on end-of-life issues? Absolutely. Should doctors be paid for providing that service? Absolutely. It adds value to health care, regardless of whatever final, end-of-life decisions a patient and family might make. Informing patients about their options, especially in the technologically and emotionally complex arena of end-of-life care – and taking the time to talk through those tough decisions with empathy – are two aspects of medicine that we as a society should agree have value.

Sound bite: "your insurance won't change"

During the debates on health reform, several politicians went on record saying that consumers could keep their current insurance if the full plan outlined in the Affordable Care Act came into effect. But given the impact of the legislation, that may not hold true. Since the federal government would cap the amount that private health insurers could put into their financial reserves, then the playing field wouldn't be level, making it hard for private insurers to compete with the unlimited pockets of federal government. A reform plan that's thousands of pages long, of course, guarantees that both proponents and opponents can spin the mandates within it one way or another to suit their own agendas.

President Obama also claimed on national television that his proposal would not in any way jeopardize people's employment benefits, and that if people currently had insurance they were happy with, they wouldn't have to change. But the eventual bill proposed new, government-run healthcare plans for people who didn't have insurance; and if employers didn't provide insurance, then their employees would be eligible to join this plan funded with federal money. If an employer didn't offer healthcare benefits to its employees, it would have to pay a penalty.

Here's the rub: The proposed penalty is only $2,000 per fulltime employee, effective January 1, 2014. That's an unrealistically low number; employers spend much more than $2,000 per employee per year to provide coverage now. The ACA calls for all employers with at least 50 fulltime employees that don't offer coverage to pay these penalties (excluding their first 30 employees from the assessment). Small companies with fewer than 50 fulltime employees are exempt.

Given skyrocketing insurance costs, many employers won't be able to afford to continue offering health benefits for their employees in the future. Hidden to most employees in their benefits packages lies their employers' costs to offer health benefits. According to the U.S. Department of Labor (DOL), the relative weight of employers' costs for employee compensation in June 2011, within private industry, was just over 70% for "wages and salaries" and just under 30% for "benefits." Of these benefits, which include vacation and retirement plans, "health benefits" carved out 7.6%. State and local governments paid even more –11.6% – of their total compensation for health benefits during the same period.

Further, in June 2011 the average private worker was paid $28.13 an hour; and out of that, 7.6% ($2.14) went to pay for medical insurance. Given that the average fulltime employee works 2,000 hours a year, that equates to $4,280 per year per employee for health care (2,000 hours multiplied by $2.14 per hour of paid-out healthcare benefit). If corporate benefits managers need to cut costs, it appears that they could hypothetically net over a 50% savings for dropping their current medical coverage and instead paying the $2,000-per-employee penalty. Note that the DOL's data of $4,280 per year per employee for health care shows the national average cost; the incentive would be even greater for companies providing higher-end, premium benefits to drop coverage.

Clearly, such a low penalty compared to high insurance costs creates a strong incentive for employers to pay the penalty and stop providing expensive medical benefits. In turn, more companies dropping their medical benefits would force workers to change their current insurance plans, even if they're happy with them. So the sound bite claiming that you can keep your current insurance without any changes that would affect your current coverage likely will prove untrue.

Other sound bites claimed that the new government-run plans would make up only a small part of the healthcare system. But the ACA virtually guarantees, given the incentives for employers to drop health insurance, that more people would migrate to the government-run plans. The penalty structure becomes an incentive that practically guarantees growing the federal program.

Democrats claimed that the healthcare reform would create a level playing field, that the new government-run program would compete fairly with the private insurers. But there's a clause in the ACA requiring that existing healthcare insurers such as Blue Cross or Regence must return any profit above 15% to the consumer. On the surface it sounds like a fine idea: Let's keep the insurance companies from becoming rich. In reality, insurance companies can only survive if they maintain a reserve that's safely invested to protect themselves financially when they make bad predictions for the year. It's part of the risk pool concept; health insurance companies have to be able to write a check when a consumer needs care. There's a big difference between insuring yourself as a consumer with a company that has $6 billion in reserve and one that has $6 million. Consumers may assume that insurers all have roughly the same level of reserves, but they actually vary; and even with regulation by the federal government, some insurance companies have gone belly-up. With the ACA legislation, private insurers would be limited by how much money they can keep in their reserve funds, but no such limits are placed on the government program. It's a given that private insurance premiums will rise due to increased costs of doing business, so the federal program would become the default program with increasing numbers of enrollees.

Political realities: looking ahead

According to the nonpartisan Kaiser Family Foundation, as of October 2011, only 34% of Americans viewed the Affordable Care Act passed in 2010 favorably. Some of the ACA mandates have become law, although given the decline in Americans' approval of the ACA since its passage, some of these mandates may eventually be adjusted to deal with political realities on the ground going forward.

Further, since most mandates in the ACA legislation haven't been funded by Congress, they're not fully in effect. In February 2011, the Republican-controlled House passed a "continuing resolution" to continue funding government programs at previous levels through September 2011, the end of the federal government's fiscal year. As of this writing, a new federal budget still hasn't been passed, which leaves full implementation of the Affordable Care Act still on the table until an overall federal budget has been set. As long as Republicans maintain power in the House, some of the legislative mandates in the proposal may be repealed. As of October 2011, support even began to drop from Democrats and voters who had previously agreed with the reform plan, putting healthcare reform in further jeopardy. Alternative measures that have been proposed, such as Health Savings Accounts, simply aren't enough to fix the fiscal healthcare crisis.

At the end of the day, if citizens need medical care but can't afford it, most Americans won't deny them care. I would argue, as most physicians and a good portion of the public would argue, that health care is a moral obligation for a developed society to provide. In all fairness to politicians, health care has become too complex an issue to resolve using sound bites, although in our media-driven culture, sound bites often rule the roost in public decision-making. So regardless of the fate of the Affordable Care Act of 2010, we as physicians don't need a prophet to read the handwriting on the wall. The healthcare crisis has not yet been resolved, and we as healthcare providers can no longer follow the crisis from the sidelines. Further change is coming, and physicians need to become more active leaders in the change to take us into the future.

CHAPTER 6
The Role of Proactive Physician Leaders

Reforming health care to become more collaborative, value-driven, and cost-effective will require a long-term, culturally sensitive point of view. Within the provider culture, the process starts with breaking down barriers and learning to practice as collaborative physicians versus maintaining an autonomous approach to care. Since healthcare costs cannot continue to approach 20% of GDP and dramatically outpace inflation, physicians can no longer afford to work in a reactive mode, imagine themselves autonomous, and avoid driving change. True, they're frustrated that Medicare cuts their reimbursement again and again, but until physicians leave that reactive, almost victimized mindset, positive change can't happen.

When it comes to physician leadership, hospitals and other healthcare organizations typically hand the ball off to their Human Resources staff, who see leadership training as their purview. Since they're not physicians themselves, HR staff may be quite unfamiliar with the physicians' culture and are likely to meet with doctors' resistance to change. The physician appointed as Chief Medical Officer may become involved, as well, in deciding whether to bring leadership training to the doctors on staff, but both CMOs and staff doctors tend to bring a mindset of "make a diagnosis and fix it immediately," which can actually hamper progress.

Physicians need to start asking, "What is realistic and could actually work for healthcare reform? In what ways can we contribute to the best solution possible given the funding on hand?" Until physician leaders in hospitals and other healthcare organizations work from that paradigm – and can communicate it consistently and positively to other physicians they work with – doctors will likely remain in a more passive, pessimistic mindset.

That's why I tell doctors in my physician leadership trainings, as Bill Gates says, that the best way to predict the future is to invent it. Change is coming, and the time to take the reins is now. Since no one understands health care as well as physicians do, they're best positioned to lead the charge, evaluate reform proposals, draft their own ideas to change the reimbursement scheme, and increase value. The clinical training of physicians puts them in an ideal position to preserve the best elements of clinical care today and lead the way toward an even better system – rather than end up, by default, with a single-party-payer model. Healthcare reform proposals should come from inside the physician community rather than primarily from the political arena.

Solutions from the ground up

The solutions in health care have to come from the ground up – providers in the trenches – by paying hospital systems a given amount of money for a set number of patients. The idea is not to micromanage these hospital systems but to have them track broad outcomes such as morbidity, mortality, access to care, and other outcomes proven by firm, nonfudgeable data. Just as airlines have safety regulations, hospital systems can have patient-safety monitoring without micromanaging and overburdening the physicians. Consumers expect quality and safety in health care, but how hospitals and doctors provide it can be – and I believe should be – left up to the providers to a large degree.

If all staff members in a hospital embraced the idea that they have a mission to serve their community in the best way possible with limited resources, they'd make sure that all of the care they provided as a group offered the greatest value. If doctors or nurses thought they could do something better, they'd be able to bring that up for discussion without being intimidated or blocked from decision-making, which would require a change in the culture of medicine and the way healthcare organizations are run.

Many hospitals are now trying to implement the "lean" culture that Toyota made famous. That process works outside of health care because the companies that implemented it became profitable once consumers evaluated their products and decided they had value: good quality and a reasonable price tag. People pay for the value of Toyota's entire product, not separately for each airbag or bumper. Successful "lean" cultures also work because of the relationship between the company and its employees, who are empowered to fix problems when they see them; they don't have to ask anyone's permission. Health care isn't that kind of collaborative culture. For methods involved in the "lean" culture to succeed in health care, physician leaders first need to change the current culture.

Determining cost-effective quality of care

To succeed, ending fee-for-service reimbursement and paying hospital and physician systems prospectively would mean letting them figure out how to provide cradle-to-grave care for a given number of patients in a certain region for a set price. The payment scheme then aligns the incentive with the mission: quality of care that's cost-effective.

In cardiology today, for example, a private practitioner can provide a good deal of care that's arbitrary. That's not a criticism; it's a reality in our tradition as cardiologists, in part because we've had no incentive to rethink the system. Cardiologists know that they'll be reimbursed more for an EKG than for the office visit when they sit and talk with the patient. That's not "high-value" medicine, especially when an EKG might not even be necessary or add value to that patient's care.

It begs the question: How do physicians know whether a given test is "medically necessary" or they can do without it? They're more likely to take the time to figure that out if they have an incentive. Over the last decade, doctors have seen much more push-back from patients, questioning whether they really need a given test, since the burden of cost has been shifting to patients through higher co-pays and co-insurance. But practically speaking, doctors are still the final decision-makers of utilization in most cases.

A patient may have an office visit co-pay of $20, for instance, which includes anything done in the office that day. So the patient may logically think, "I'm already here, I've paid my $20, so give me everything you've got to be on the safe side." Clearly, with procedures like cardiac catheterization that have larger co-insurance, patients ask more questions about whether they really need them. But when a physician is adamant about the need for a procedure, the overwhelming majority of patients will agree to have it done. Similarly, if a doctor feels comfortable that a procedure isn't needed, most patients who trust that doctor will agree to forgo it. So when some doctors today complain that patients are coming in "demanding" this and "demanding" that, it reveals as much about the physician culture as the patients' actual mindset. Most patients don't really demand anything; they're coming into the office to ask questions and have a discussion, looking for a peer-to-peer relationship rather than an authoritative one.

When doctors aren't prepared for that kind of conversation, they can interpret it negatively. As physicians, they're trained to resist being challenged and, frankly, to fight back; they're trained that way in medical school and even more so in residency. Physicians are very expensively and very well trained to be the purveyors of knowledge, the ultimate authority. That's the indoctrinated image: being in charge and knowing more than someone else in the face of a challenge. That intensely competitive mindset, especially in academic medicine, will eventually disappear with the right physician leadership training, but we can't wait for it to die out by attrition. The healthcare crisis can't wait that long.

Not "gatekeeping" but resource management

The idea of doctors as "gatekeepers" arose in the 1980s as a key component in HMOs and managed care and was marketed to consumers as a positive benefit: your primary care doctor as your source for deciding the best treatment for you. Primary care physicians received a "capitated" payment of a certain number of dollars per member per month. They spent money caring for the patient out of this payment; any money left over went to the primary care doctor as compensation.

Gatekeeping was based on the assumption that healthcare costs were driven by specialty care, and that if primary care doctors were incentivized to use specialty care less, overall healthcare costs would drop. That assumption didn't take into account why specialty care costs more. It's not because specialists charge more to see a patient than primary care docs do; it's that the reimbursement system drives specialists to overutilize expensive technology, and it's the overuse of that expensive technology that's driving healthcare costs. Gatekeeping could only control costs by denying people access to specialty care since overall patient care was not integrated or capitated. Nobody's advocating gatekeeping anymore, especially not politicians seeking reelection.

Instead, I'm calling for a closer look at quality and figuring out the most cost-effective way to provide it – that is, defining value. With national costs in mind, then, if a consumer chooses a more expensive model of care without demonstrable improvement in quality, he or she should pay for the difference. If penicillin is the safe, effective drug of choice for pneumococcal pneumonia but a patient demands the newest, most expensive drug, then that patient should pay the difference for that drug.

Only physicians have the training and expertise to step back and take a broader look at the entire system to use medical resources more wisely. If a healthcare organization with primary care doctors, specialists, and inpatient and outpatient facilities were all incentivized to work together by receiving a fixed amount of money every year, that organization would figure out how best to use their specialists and primary care doctors; those facilities would design innovative ways of delivering care that would be consistent and offer high value. The idea is not to deny patients the ability to see specialists; the idea is to be clear on what the specialists can offer to individuals – and offer to the system. If specialists spend time developing protocols that primary care doctors can use, for instance, and those protocols assure patients they're receiving the best care, that's not gatekeeping and it's not denying care – it's wise resource management in medicine.

Once again it comes back to fee-for-service reimbursement and the need to stop paying specialists more to use technology, and instead pay them to work together with primary care doctors and facilities to take care of patients. When specialists, instead, are incentivized to order and interpret MRIs, perform cardiac catheterizations, or surgically implant stents and prosthetic devices, a huge financial demand is placed on overall healthcare costs. Current incentives focus on quantity, not value.

In a clinically driven reform of the system that eliminates fee-for-service, we'd ask specialists how they're going to make sure that every patient who receives expensive technology actually needs it. Even more important: Whether a specialist does thousands of procedures or does only one, it wouldn't make any difference in that physician's income or improve the organization's bottom line. Eliminating fee-for-service would eliminate the inherent conflicts of interest and incentives to use expensive technology, which would then only be used for a patient's benefit, not a physician's. The focus changes from quantity of reimbursement to quality and value of care for patients.

Physician integration to reduce costs

Rarely do primary care doctors and specialists work together collaboratively and noncompetitively because of the turf wars going on today. Many physicians are competitive by nature; that is, after all, how we made it into medical school. But there are fewer turf wars in integrated healthcare systems than in private practice. In successfully integrated systems – when they include both primary and specialty care physicians – the physicians have figured out when to refer a patient to a specialist or not, and how to utilize their specialists in the most "high-value" way. Integrated delivery systems have improved the relationship between specialists and primary care doctors because they're all working together, even if they have complicated formulas for reimbursement. When systems are integrated and doctors are incentivized the right way, they can determine the best interaction between primary and specialty care better than nonclinicians.

We probably need more primary care doctors and fewer specialists than we currently have, but doctors and delivery systems could figure that out themselves if the fee-for-service incentives disappear. If we start integrating health care and find out that a large percentage of procedures are unnecessary, then medical school programs will naturally produce fewer proceduralists to match that lower need. The market can figure that out; every physician who's trained to do procedures starts their training as general physicians, so if doctors find they're not needed as proceduralists, they can start seeing patients in the office. Instead of having government agencies micromanage this, providers can sort this out. The first step in this process is an overhaul of reimbursement.

While physicians don't go into medicine to become entrepreneurs, every professional is a creature of economic reality. If physicians find a group that will pay more for their services, they may decide to work exclusively for that group, even if the work isn't as fun or challenging. Physicians haven't intentionally set about to tweak the system to make as much money as possible, but the system has given them economic incentives to do so – and disincentives to do otherwise. If we're paying physicians 20 or 30 times more to do a procedure than to talk with a patient, what's the natural human response to this in a competitive market? On the other hand, if physicians made no extra money doing procedures, what would be the consequences? Some physicians argue that it wouldn't change their utilization behavior at all; that's a natural moral stance, but in reality some physicians' utilization behavior might change. Certainly, the specialty procedure utilization rates at integrated delivery systems such as the U.S. Veterans Affairs hospital systems, Group Health in Seattle, or Kaiser Permanente in California are lower than they are at nonintegrated hospitals.

An international comparison of utilization patterns also illustrates the point that fee-for-service drives the use of resources. For many countries, utilization rates are dictated by governments who tell providers what they'll pay each year for health care; when the money runs out, that's it. Curiously, even in a system like that – anathema to many Americans used to no limits on health care – their longevity statistics aren't worse than ours, but often better. The United States ranked 48th in longevity in 2011, with a life expectancy of 78.37 years, falling behind Canada and all of Western Europe. A study published in *Population Health Metrics* comparing health status and health-related quality of life between the United States and Canada showed no overall differences except in low-income people, where the Canadians actually fared better. The data shows that while it's difficult to compare countries and their spending, it's disingenuous to assume that the marked increase in U.S. healthcare spending provides measurably better outcomes. When we look at value – quality divided by cost – there is clearly room for improvement in the United States.

Beyond fragmentation: a continuum of care

A more integrated system offering a continuum of care would cut overutilization of expensive resources as well as address the problems caused by medical care that has become fragmented, chaotic, and episodic. Physician leaders can be invaluable in redesigning elements of the care continuum to address the clinical issues and unnecessary expenses incurred with such fragmented care.

If you have high blood pressure, for example, and you have good health insurance, your doctor may ask you to come into the office to have your blood pressure checked every three months. But checking your blood pressure every three months in an office has little to do with your actual, daily blood pressure. A better, more cost-effective solution might be for you to learn to check your own blood pressure at home, with a caregiver to teach you how, review your blood pressure reports, and monitor your progress. You could do this at home and report in online, instead of paying for an office visit with an expensive provider every three months. Physicians could develop clear algorithms for less-expensive caregivers to implement, such as weekly calls to patients, checking on weekly blood pressure readings, and monitoring patients' reports to the doctor through a secure website for privacy. Only if a patient's blood pressure rose above given levels more than twice a week would he or she need to come into the office and incur those costs.

Another example: Patients with congestive heart failure may go home from the hospital with 20 medications, when their medicine cabinet at home is already overflowing with medications, some of which duplicate what they're taking home from the hospital. The "medication reconciliation" process during discharge from the hospital, trying to get all the medications straight before sending the patient home, rarely works well because many patients can't remember what they have at home. So when a congestive heart failure patient leaves the hospital, a value-driven, continuum-of-care model might include sending a low-cost care provider out to the patient's home the next day to do an inventory of the medicine cabinet, organize their medications in labeled pill boxes, and make it easy for the patient to take their medications correctly and safely.

These caregivers may or may not even have a college degree; the point is that they're trained to follow physician-designed algorithms to extend cost-effective care into the home. They offer the added benefit of all the information they're gathering once they walk in the home; they can tell if patients aren't taking good care of themselves and can flag those patients as "at risk," and perhaps visit with at-risk patients more frequently for monitoring. The goal is an inexpensive solution to extend care: not a physician, not a registered nurse, but a less expensive, hourly home health employee. This model could extend care into the wellness arena, as well, such as to make sure heart failure patients are weighing themselves regularly, ask what they're eating, check up on salt consumption, and otherwise monitor their overall health. No matter how it's framed in buzzwords – "wellness" or "continuum of care" – extending low-cost care into the home could help patients take better care of themselves and manage chronic diseases with high-value healthcare delivery models.

Integrated systems: value and cost control

An integrated healthcare system that looks closely at cost control, in both physicians' and consumers' minds, often carries a negative association with the idea that those systems withhold care. Yet their outcomes data doesn't suggest that. In a study of patients with end-stage renal disease, for instance, investigators compared care at Southern California Kaiser-Permanente, a large, self-insured, integrated healthcare system, with traditional fee-for-service care. The study found several unique features of the Kaiser-Permanente approach to managing kidney disease. Kaiser doctors routinely screen their patients for renal disease to increase early detection. Patients with kidney disease are treated by multidisciplinary teams that include a nephrologist, renal case manager, renal dietician, renal social worker, and renal pharmacist, with a team leader who communicates a shared vision, fosters teamwork focused on patient care, and decides how to allocate patient-care resources. Nephrologists serve as salaried primary care physicians, with dialysis provided onsite. The team uses disease management protocols that focus on maintaining kidney function; managing comorbid conditions such as hypertension and diabetes; managing vascular access (for example, protecting a patient's dominant arm from IV lines and blood drawing); and modifying lifestyle with weight control, smoking cessation, and exercise.

The investigators found several differences in outcomes between Kaiser and traditional Medicare fee-for-service patients. Kaiser patients were seen by kidney specialists earlier in the disease process, as well as more regularly throughout the course of illness, than were the traditional fee-for-service patients. Only half of the end-stage renal disease patients at Kaiser had not seen a nephrologist in their pre-end-stage renal disease timeframe, while nearly three-quarters of fee-for-service patients had not seen a nephrologist during that time.

Further, in the year prior to and first year after the onset of end-stage renal disease, Kaiser patients used fewer hospital days compared with fee-for-service patients. Kaiser patients used an average of 12 hospital days during the year prior to onset and 17 hospital days one year afterward, while fee-for-service patients used 16.6 hospital days during the year prior to onset and 28.2 hospital days during the year after onset. Even after the researchers controlled for other factors that could contribute to hospital use, such as diabetes and cardiovascular conditions, these differences in the data persisted.

In some of the earlier models of integrated facilities such as Group Health, accessibility was an issue, and if you had a medical problem, there could often be a delay in seeing a doctor – with access to specialists even more controlled. Access remains an open question in healthcare reform; putting controls on seeing doctors and specialists carries with it both pros and cons. When Medicare has to investigate a cardiologist who appears to have implanted 585 medically unnecessary stents, having a few more controls on access looks like a good idea. As a physician, I would argue that we'd be better off with a handful of integrated delivery systems such as Kaiser or Group Health, staffed with skilled physician leadership deciding on care and determining fees, rather than a single-party-payer system.

Creating new payment paradigms

The sustainable growth rate formula designed to control physician reimbursement, tied to Medicare when the federal balanced budget amendment was passed in 1997, carries with it a fundamental problem: trying to control costs with an across-the-board slashing of physician reimbursement. But the rate at which doctors are paid is not the issue; it isn't that physicians charge too much money to see patients in the office. The real issue is that physicians have been financially forced to make up for declining income by increasing procedures that will reimburse them, which clearly drives up national utilization of expensive resources. So until we fix the payment *paradigm* – not the *rate* – by which doctors are reimbursed, healthcare costs will continue to spiral out of control.

In fact, increasing reimbursement for what we want physicians to do – such as primary care medicine and working on revamping the system to create more value – would be more effective than the across-the-board cuts we're doing now.

In the past there was a push from Medicare and private insurers toward "pay for performance," and they're still talking about it now. In fact, the idea of "paying for performance" plays a central role in the Accountable Care Organization (ACO) concept and how doctors can play a key, positive role in ACO development. But American health care has already been paying for performance; we've just been paying for the wrong kind of performance. We're getting exactly what we're paying for by tagging incentives on high-ticket procedures. Payers see the issue, but they're met with tremendous resistance when they try to change the paradigm by which they reimburse; it's been much easier for them to change the rates. The discussion ends up focusing on the wrong issue. The primary issue is that health care costs too much because of overutilization, and it can't be solved by decreasing the *rate* of reimbursement. It can't be emphasized enough: Reimbursement is not the issue; overutilization is the issue.

Some experts suggest that the solution is to salary all physicians, but those salaries would still be fed by a system that bills in a fee-for-service mode. Until payers like Medicare, Medicaid, and private insurers change their paradigm of paying for care and eliminate fee-for-service, national costs won't ever change significantly.

The prospective payment system for Medicare was a good idea and has likely slowed the rate of growth in healthcare spending, although policy experts argue over the specific amount of likely savings. It has certainly forced hospitals to analyze more closely how they're providing care and try to cut some "fat" from their systems, but because of waivers to the sustainable growth rates and adding codes to DRGs to increase their reimbursements, providers have found ways to circumvent the ultimate purpose of the prospective payment model, which was to control costs.

Physician-driven protocols to control costs

Every physician could come up with a multitude of low-cost ways to provide better quality care and improve healthcare value. For patients with congestive heart failure, for instance, where daily fluctuations of body weight can signal a potentially serious problem requiring medical attention, the care team could ask: Does the patient have a scale at home? If not, perhaps the integrated system should buy one; it might save money in the long run. Do patients have a working phone at home so they can call the doctor if they have a problem, and a working pair of glasses so they can read the names on their prescriptions? Can they hear accurately, or do they need a hearing aid?

Other examples of improving patient care: Physicians often discharge elderly patients from the hospital with a follow-up visit scheduled in one, two, or three weeks after they're sent home, depending on physicians' schedules. It could be that long before many patients come in contact with the healthcare system again. It's unfortunate, it's typical, but it's not optimal quality of care.

With elderly patients, what are the chances that they understand everything providers tell them as they leave the hospital? Zip. They've been in the strange hospital environment, they're stressed out and confused, and many of them aren't thinking or remembering clearly in that environment. Some of them are scared to death because they're leaving the hospital where competent caregivers are nearby around the clock, and they're going home where they'll be with untrained family members or, worse, they'll be alone.

A physician tells those elderly patients as they leave the hospital, "This medicine is the same as this medicine, and the red pill is the same as the green pill, which is also the same as the blue pill; but don't take all three together. Make sure you take this one with food, but this one, don't take with food; and take this one at night, but make sure you don't take this one at night; and by the way don't take these two together, ever. Okay, we'll see you in two weeks." You have to wonder what's happening to elderly patients at home during those first few weeks, confused and trying to take their medications correctly.

The home health model, for instance, where a home health worker goes into the home and checks in with patients on a regular basis following hospitalization, has proved successful by many standards. But today, home health services aren't automatic; they must be ordered by a doctor and aren't typically part of an integrated delivery system. Only patients declared in need of those services are tracked in the system, and home health reimbursement resides in its own "silo," separate from other medical costs. Clearly, if all medical services, from surgery to home health, were part of an integrated system of patient care – both delivery of care and payment of care – costs could be more easily tracked and controlled. Doctors could then view home health care not as a competitive loss for themselves but as an overall gain, since it would reduce the number of expensive physician visits, lower overall costs, maintain quality of care, and reward all providers in the system.

More physician leaders should be thinking "outside of the box" about how to improve care while still controlling costs. If patients with chronic diseases such as congestive heart failure, for example, can do well at home without repeated hospitalizations, an integrated system saves a lot of money – funds that could be spent monitoring patients at home while still being profitable as a system. Hospitalizations are expensive for everyone: the hospital, the patient, and the country's healthcare system. Patients have a continuum of needs that can be met by a continuum of people on a continuum of pay scales. What would be the cost ramifications, for instance, if patients received a daily call from a trained caregiver after hospitalization to help them keep their medications sorted out, someone not necessarily as well trained and expensive as a registered nurse? A few integrated delivery systems have looked at the costs and benefits of a similar algorithm; it's worth looking at on a larger scale.

Physicians understand these practical issues because they see what happens to patient care and outcomes when these issues aren't being addressed. Unfortunately, there's currently no incentive for physicians to fix these clinical issues; in fact, there's a subliminal disincentive since more patients then slip through the cracks and end up back in the care of physicians who can charge them in the fee-for-service model. Physicians would realize the benefits even more in an integrated system with prospective payments because it would more directly affect the bottom line.

One well-respected, successful Seattle hospital, for instance, has developed a back pain protocol that has saved millions of dollars. Every time a patient arrives with a back problem, the staff follows this protocol. The patient is first seen not by a doctor but by a physical therapist, who does a complete back evaluation and decides what needs to be done for that patient. The team has avoided unnecessary surgeries, had better outcomes, and saved considerable amounts of money in today's fee-for-service model. If they had been paid prospectively for those patients, they would likely have saved even more.

This hospital used its protocol despite the fact that it could be "losing money" by ordering fewer surgeries and MRIs. Their leadership wanted to evaluate the potential for savings, knowing that the national system is heading in the direction of bundled payments. Despite the initial fears of financial loss, the hospital actually saved money because the total volume of MRIs decreased, so they avoided having to buy a new MRI scanner. Their patients saved money since they avoided co-pays for surgery, unnecessary hospitalizations, and being out of work – and, most importantly, they had measurably better outcomes.

Physicians as change agents

Here's the rub. When a local hospital leader talks about an operational idea that produces great results, other administrators often make a note, thinking they'll go back to their own hospitals to try it. But does that mean they're able to implement the new program? Probably not. Back at their hospitals, they likely meet with push-back from their doctors, particularly the ones with the most to lose in making some sort of change, such as revising their clinical pathways to match those of their successful colleagues' or letting go of fee-for-service.

That's where physician leadership comes in. Change happens with leaders who have a vision, remain true to the vision and communicate it well, hold people accountable, and keep moving forward. Some healthcare organizations have had problems with physician turnover while trying to gain control over costs; that's the common fall-out when leadership starts pushing the vision of "Toyota lean" or other proven value-driven programs. To control costs, the staff at those hospitals has had to buy into the idea that medicine is better when it's more consistently practiced and delivered with less variation.

Hospitalists: a case of physician-generated change

The birth of the hospitalist specialty exemplifies how physicians can drive healthcare process improvement in cooperation with their hospitals. After large group practices had hired a lot of primary care physicians back in the 1980s, they found that their physicians were inefficient, driving back and forth to the hospital to see their own patients. The physician leaders running the primary care clinics saw a better way to do things, more efficient and profitable for the group as a whole: They created hospitalists.

No agency mandated the creation of hospitalists. Instead, these large medical groups in primary care began looking at their own efficiency and designating a few internal medicine and family doctors they'd rotate into the hospital as the "hospital doctor" for that month. It was a "reform from within," driven by physicians, and a great idea, both in terms of quality of hospital care and overall efficiency of the healthcare system.

Efficiency is often a byproduct of specialization, and the new specialty, the hospitalists, became specialists in managing inpatient care. They evolved as in-house specialists in caring for patients during a hospital stay, to coordinate their specialty and subspecialty care, diagnostic testing, surgery, pharmacy, and other hospital resources those inpatients need. I was a practicing cardiologist during this change; we at Northwest Hospital were among the first community hospitals in Seattle to have hospitalists practicing in our facility, beginning in the 1990s. Part of my job at the time as ICU Director was to go out into the physician community and convince the primary care doctors who referred to our hospital that this was going to work – that it wouldn't be a threat to their practices. Primary care doctors were worried that their patients would never come back to them for their medical care, that patients would somehow be persuaded to keep seeing the hospitalist responsible for their care in the hospital.

One of our solutions was to hire hospitalists who had no offices themselves; they only worked in our hospital, which made them less of a threat to the referring physicians. I sold the idea to primary care doctors by reminding them that instead of driving to the hospital and back to their offices, losing two hours of the day without reimbursement, they could see patients back in the office and survive financially. It was initially an economically driven decision, but hospitalists with attention to and control over the communication process – from the hospital back to primary care physicians – also improve overall patient care.

Our hospital decided to hire several nurse practitioners to work with the hospitalists to coordinate communication back to the primary care physicians. Every referring physician identified a preferred method of communication: Some wanted to receive phone calls every morning with the clinical update on each of their patients; others wanted their updates faxed or emailed; still others had nurses designated to receive the communication. We made sure that primary care physicians received an update every day about their patients in the hospital and received a phone call about any significant change, so they were reassured that they weren't cut out of any communication loops. The attention to communication and collaboration helped the transition and integration of a new specialty in the system work well. It's this understanding of both the clinical and operational nuances that will make future, ground-up reform successful in health care.

The bottom line in the hospital: Patients fare much better when there's a team around all the time. Instead of a hospital nurse having to pick up the phone and call a patient's primary care doctor in the middle of a busy office day and wait for the doctor to make it to the phone to order a test or medication change, it now happens much more quickly. With hospitalists in place, the hospital team responds immediately and care moves along more efficiently. From the hospital's point of view, hiring in-house hospitalists is also a cost-saving strategy to help control the utilization of expensive hospital resources.

Medicine has developed to the point of nuance and sophistication where "Dr. Welby" has disappeared. Clinical care has become so specialized that physicians can't excel at seeing patients in the office and also have that same level of comfort and skill around critically ill patients in the hospital. Similarly, intensive care specialists don't have the same outpatient skills and talents as primary care physicians who diagnose a wide breadth of patients all day.

The general level of disease severity in the hospital has also changed; patients today are rarely admitted to the hospital unless they're extremely ill. The system is doing a better job of preventing unnecessary hospital stays by providing more care in outpatient settings such as an office or clinic. But now that medical technology has made outpatient clinical care more available, nearly every patient who ends up in the hospital needs highly sophisticated – and therefore more expensive – intensive care. For all these reasons, hospitalists are a step in the right direction toward improving quality of care, and they're here to stay due to the economic realities of hospital reimbursement.

More cases of physician-driven change

Using intensivists (doctors who specialize in intensive care medicine) is another positive, physician-driven initiative shown to improve care and reduce costs in intensive care units. The Leapfrog Group, a voluntary initiative among Fortune 500 companies to evaluate hospital care and costs, now rates around-the-clock availability of intensivists as an essential factor in a hospital's ability to provide quality care.

The rise of advanced registered nurse practitioners (ARNPs) and physician assistants (PAs) is another physician-driven change that has been successful. When physicians evaluated how they were spending their time, they realized they could fare better financially if they had medically qualified staff working for them; again, specialization often leads to greater efficiency and profitability. Initially, physicians began using nurse practitioners and PAs not as independent practitioners but as auxiliary members of their teams. The open-heart surgeons at Providence Hospital in Seattle, for instance, hired nurse practitioners back in the 1980s to perform most of the post-operative care for them, so surgeons could stay in the OR, do more surgeries, and know that their patients were being well taken care of after surgery. The surgeons became much more productive. Other physicians use nurse practitioners to dictate hospital discharge summaries; the ARNPs, who don't feel the same time crunch that physicians do to rush out of the hospital and back to their offices to see patients, often do a better job dictating in the absence of those time pressures.

The rise of congestive heart failure clinics illustrates another example of physician-generated change to improve quality of care and become more efficient from the ground up. These clinics bring together a team of doctors, nurses, social workers, and aides to coordinate the care of critically ill patients across the continuum of care, thereby decreasing errors, costs, and hospital readmissions for this expensive, chronically ill patient population. These examples prove how physician-driven change, determined by physicians and other clinicians working well together and collaborating on the ground, can achieve better outcomes – even if, as with many changes in health care, the initial impetus is financial.

A case of MD leadership: safety protocols

When I recently went to a Seattle hospital for a shoulder injection, I came in contact with more than a dozen different staff, each of whom asked for my full name and date of birth. Consumers might think that's annoying, but there's a good reason why they're doing it: to make sure they have the right patient getting the right procedure. Medical errors with patients do occasionally happen, but even one is unacceptable.

This same hospital had been the setting for one well-publicized case years ago, when a physician made a critical mistake in a radiology suite with an injection that caused a patient death. Instead of glossing it over, the hospital CEO, a forward-thinking physician leader, went to the family and apologized, and talked with everyone in the hospital system about what had happened and how they could prevent it from happening again, by working together to fix everything that had gone wrong. The CEO didn't take away the hospital privileges of the physician in error or fire the nurse who handed him the wrong vial – although those are common responses – and instead decided to find out how the system could have allowed it to happen. He then challenged everyone on staff to embrace new safety protocols with increased checks and balances to ensure that a similar mistake wouldn't happen again.

Hence the dozen or so check-points with staff who repeatedly checked my name and date of birth. Today, their protocols ensure that each patient matches up to the right diagnosis and the right drug or procedure. It may be tedious to experience as a consumer, but airline pilots and copilots do the same thing in the cockpit: Checking and re-checking details over again, together, is what safety is all about.

Physician culture change

Because a significantly collaborative hospital culture would represent a significant change for physicians, it highlights the need for physician leaders. It's a complete paradigm shift for doctors to become part of a cooperative corporate culture instead of thinking and working as autonomous, independent practitioners. Physicians tend to rebel against standardization, so there's push-back when hospital leaders tell their doctors, "When you see each patient, you must verify the date of birth," or "You can't inject anything until it's been checked by the nurse in the lab or the radiation tech." It's a minefield any time hospitals try to standardize, given the resistance they meet from their staff physicians. When hospitals decide that they can't afford to stock 20 different stents and can stock only 10, for instance, physicians push back, even when there's no solid evidence that the 10 nonstocked stents perform any better than the rest.

Adopting new electronic medical record systems is another prime example of the need for physicians to drop their mindset of autonomy and adapt to today's changing medical culture. The technology for "computerized physician order entry" (CPOE) has been available for several years, and the need for it has been documented by every entity in the playing field that scores hospital quality. The Joint Commission, the Institute for Healthcare Improvement, the Leapfrog Group, and others have all recognized CPOE as an indicator of quality and have pushed hospitals to institute it. Hospital leaders have invested in their infrastructure and spent a fortune on new computer hardware and software, because none of their old hospital computers supported CPOE. It's been a bonanza for IT companies nationwide, but to this day, only a small minority of hospitals has successfully instituted computerized physician order entry.

Why? The healthcare IT systems currently on the market have been regulation-driven, first by the need for electronic billing and more recently to comply with the push for CPOE. They haven't been designed with the end user – the physician – in mind. Doctors don't want to use the new systems; it takes too much extra time. CPOE systems require physicians to type in their patient-care orders on a keyboard rather than simply handwriting their notes. Even more onerous to the physicians' autonomy: Some of the software systems direct doctors through a series of questions they have to answer before moving to each new screen to ensure that what they're ordering is safe. If physicians order a nonstandard drug or nonstandard dose, the software may ask questions about why they're doing it – flying directly in the face of physicians' training toward autonomy.

In the past, hospitals gave physicians an order sheet, sometimes simply a checklist, for their "physician orders." As a practicing cardiologist, it used to take me less than a minute to fill out an order sheet, no matter how complicated the patient's situation was; all of us physicians were in the habit of doing it that way. With CPOE, you have to sign in to a computer with your password and change your password frequently for security. CPOE software is safety-focused, not physician-focused; it wasn't designed with physicians' busy realities or psychology in mind. It's an obstacle for time-stressed doctors already deluged with new procedures, new technology, and new office billing codes, adding more administrative hurdles to an already stressful, time-crunched day. So physician resistance is understandable – if ultimately untenable in the face of certain mandated operational changes in hospitals.

Leadership means motivating people to change behavior for the greater good. In the case of CPOE, at some point hospital leaders simply need to tell their doctors, "It's time; we're doing it." The Joint Commission can't mandate that it happen immediately; buying new technology, installing it, and training all staff could easily take a year. But from the hospitals' perspective, they want it rolled out as soon as possible; they've already spent as much as $10 or $11 million on a new CPOE system and don't want it sitting around unused. The Leapfrog Group and other industry "raters" continue to award hospitals high points in their grading systems for having CPOE, further contributing to the need to convince doctors to get onboard and adapt to a new system. Physician leaders, sensitive to clinical realities, are best positioned to motivate staff doctors to make these kinds of operational changes and implement them successfully.

The cultural transformation taking place in health care is unstoppable, so the question now and in the future becomes: Who's going to drive the transformation? Will it be bureaucrats who know little about health care, or will it be doctors? If physicians were in charge and you told them, "You won't be reimbursed if you don't have CPOE," they'd figure out how to have it in place tomorrow. But the hospital is at risk now, not the physicians, and most healthcare delivery systems haven't integrated the two. The orthopedist, cardiologist, and pulmonologist at a hospital haven't lost patients because the hospital hasn't implemented CPOE, so they don't see the downside to continuing to do things the old way – their way.

Any change is stressful, but changes mandated by someone else, especially when they make your life more difficult or tedious and offer no apparent upside, give you even more reason to resist. CPOE remains one of countless examples of physicians' reluctance to change clinical behavior that no longer serves today's healthcare environment, further ammunition for the need for physician leaders to work with resistant colleagues to meet the changing demands of medicine and smooth the transition toward the future.

Framing the capitation conversation

Framing the discussion of capitated payments with physicians is critical; shaping the question will shape the response. A physician might ask other doctors, "Do you want capitation and prepayment for taking care of patients?" The majority of primary care doctors would likely answer "yes," and the overwhelming majority of specialty doctors would say "no," although more specialists now recognize that the end is near for fee-for-service. By contrast, a physician leader might say to doctors, "Capitation is coming, so would you rather let the government set your rates or figure it out among your colleagues?" Framing the question this way motivates physicians to step up to the plate and become more involved in the realities of reform.

Capitation seems to be gradually coming in through the back door. When Medicare tried capitation in the past, it became a gatekeeping maneuver that kept patients from receiving care, which ultimately led to its demise. But capitation done the right way – with bundled payments, an integrated system, and physician leadership – could work.

Consider advances in basic science when initial experiments failed; instead of abandoning new ideas, persistent people kept working on them. Healthcare reform is similar. The first round of capitation from Medicare and private insurers deepened the divide between primary care and specialists, since the capitated money went to primary care doctors, who controlled how and when they were going to use specialists. Because there was no discussion with the specialists about how fees could be fairly shared, it was a disaster. In addition, since the incentive was to limit rather than revamp care, it wasn't a viable system.

Physician leaders of the future need to be willing to take the risk of managing incoming healthcare dollars and becoming as creative and collaborative as possible as they evaluate everything their team does, decide what's "fat" versus "meat," and save the "meat." When hospital systems bite the bullet and ask doctors to work more efficiently and collaboratively in this way, some staff physicians will inevitably leave the hospital and decide they'll practice their own autonomous style of medicine somewhere else. Options still exist for a more independent style of practice, but those options are starting to disappear as our country moves toward more cost-efficient, integrated models of care. Given the massive inefficiencies in the national system, if government essentially takes over health care, the current inefficiencies will seem trivial. Inefficiencies in health care cost tremendous amounts of money. Huge sums could be saved by cutting waste and "fat" – and no one knows how to cut the "fat" in medicine better than doctors.

Building a culture of communication

Patient care clearly improves with optimal communication among all members of a medical team, especially for the communication between the nurses evaluating patients directly and the attending physicians with overall responsibility for patient outcomes. Fortunately, the majority of physicians can respond quickly and amicably to a problem if a nurse has to call them at three in the morning. But it's surprising how much damage a few difficult physicians can do, even if it's a minority of doctors, when they're untrained in how teams ought to work. If they're angry with a night nurse who calls with a question, eventually that nurse stops calling even when there's a problem, leading to a negative, self-perpetuating cycle of nurse turnover and inexperienced nurses working where experienced nurses used to be. Ultimately, patient care could be compromised. Instead, in a culture of communication, nurses and other staff would feel free to question doctors, contributing to a system of checks and balances. Patients benefit when clinicians communicate openly and collaboratively about treatment.

Curiously, when doctors work in their own offices, most manage their staffs well. They know the limits of their incomes per year and their fixed costs to be in practice: office nurses, technology, rent, utilities, and front desk staff. They understand when it's appropriate to buy a new piece of equipment or refurbish the old one for another year, and they know very well what staff turnover means; it's a disaster for them. They have clear incentives to treat their own staffs with respect, but working at a hospital, where someone else is paying staff salaries and responsible for managing them, teamwork and communication can fall by the wayside and become someone else's problem.

Changing physicians' styles of thinking

Given that changing the physician culture will take time, how do we get there from here? We need a multitargeted solution that begins with changing traditional physicians' styles of thinking, which in turn starts with revamping the way medical schools train doctors.

As physicians, it can be extremely difficult to appreciate how fully our perspectives have been formed by medical indoctrination; some physicians don't realize it until they've been retired for several years. As the CEO of a large healthcare system once said to me, it's a kind of brainwashing: The physician mindset becomes so engrained and integrated into your thinking and personality that eventually it becomes invisible to you. Medicine has a long tradition, one that will be hard to change, with both honorable and limiting features. Many physicians recognize that medical training and medicine have to change, but they can be blind to how their own thinking can handicap them, prevent them from embracing change, and keep them from becoming more effective as clinicians and leaders.

Physicians are rigorously trained in a specific style of thinking: There's a problem, therefore there's a solution, and the solution can be found by reading the literature. The idea that the solution could be found within – that there are new ways they could learn to think and communicate that enhance their ability to be effective – tends to be overlooked.

That's why the leadership development process can't be rushed, especially within the physician culture; it's a time-intensive process that involves new forms of education and interaction. Ultimately, leadership development works best by coaching and mentoring physicians on an ongoing basis until they've fully integrated new ways of thinking, communicating, and interacting. Hospital CMOs may have problems they want fixed immediately, but developing physician leaders for the future requires a change toward long-term thinking at all levels of a healthcare organization, including those at the top.

Projecting costs for the future

As healthcare analysts try to project for the future, a crucial aspect of reform should be to ask what our country needs to be healthy in the future, given our population, common diseases, and the medical personnel and technology available to us. Do we have the data to look at actual health trends and outcomes as well as utilization? Why keep building projections on overutilization patterns instead of developing a minimal, workable standard of care for the future?

Part of the equation of successful reform would be to understand what's actually going on in various communities. How many people actually visited the ED? How many had heart attacks? How many people are moving into each community? How can we project the country's real needs over the next 50 to 100 years to decide what new technologies and services make the most sense – meaning they provide the best value? Projections for future healthcare spending that are based on past GDP percentages don't separate out real medical needs from past overutilization; that model only tracks what we *have been* spending, not what we *should be* spending for the best overall national outcomes for the future. Looking at projections based on past costs leads to a flawed analysis; we're already spending more than we ought to. Our healthcare financing systems have had no control over past costs, so to take uncontrolled costs and project them further would lead to a nightmare.

Conversations about capital allocations in a hospital boardroom usually focus on what a given capital expenditure will do to increase market share – versus what it will do to improve the quality of care. The problem now is hospitals are spending too much money trying to increase market share, increase payer mix, and increase profitability – that's become the game.

Who's in the best position to evaluate whether a procedure is needed and has value or not? The clinicians trained in that specialty. If you asked me as a cardiologist to think about everything I did in the office in a typical week and decide what we could eliminate because it added no clear value, I could find a handful of things right off the bat. Further, if you asked me to do that periodically, and to empower my staff to do the same kind of evaluation, the effects would be geometric. The front office staff might decide to have patients schedule their own appointments online; it would free them up to answer patients' questions when they first arrive. A nurse might realize that the same patients keep coming back to the office because they're not sure what medications to take, and it would be more cost-effective and easier for everyone if the nurse called those patients at home to check up on their medications.

Rethinking hospital marketing

Health care as an industry generates marketing concepts that become trends. Ten years ago, most large hospitals were building a "center of excellence," and suddenly every hospital became a center of excellence. More recently, the buzz around "patient-centered care" has created a way for hospitals to market their services and differentiate themselves from their competition. Hospitals want to make sure patients are happy and refer their family and friends when they need care. Focusing on the patient experience isn't a bad idea, but it doesn't change the overall drivers of cost or improve our national health.

Just as customers assume that all airlines are roughly the same with regard to safety, the initial assumption by patients when they enter a hospital system is that there's little difference in safety and quality. The way for providers to differentiate themselves in the market is by creating value, which by definition addresses the issues of safety and quality. Creating value requires changing the way we pay for health care and ending fee-for-service by putting physician leaders, not bureaucrats or politicians, in charge of an overall budget and letting them lead their colleagues in transforming the way we deliver care.

Hospitals now market themselves to consumers by focusing on the patients' experience and "hotel-like" amenities, but with little focus on cost and value. Patients are choosing a hospital based on preferences like food and how nice someone sounds on the phone. Granted, those factors are part of the quality and value model, but only a minor part.

A tragic example: My uncle, diagnosed with esophageal cancer, planned to have surgery at a small hospital around the corner from his home near Philadelphia. Esophageal cancer is a complicated disease, and the surgery is horrific. At that time, only a handful of U.S. surgeons really knew how to do it. One of the experts happened to be in downtown Philadelphia, less than a half-hour away, so I called him, and he agreed to evaluate my uncle and do the surgery. When I called the family back the next day, my uncle was already in surgery in the small, local hospital; the family hadn't wanted to go to the downtown hospital because it was "too far away" and the food was "terrible." My uncle died three weeks later from a poorly performed operation. It's a tragic story that unfortunately happens all too frequently. From the hospitals' perspective, marketing with ideas such as "patient comfort" and "convenience" makes sense in the short term to garner a larger market share, but not in the long-term picture of healthcare reform and quality of care.

Let's look instead at a new model based on prospective payment: Two hypothetical hospitals are competing for local patients on a per-patient, per-year payment scheme. A local insurance company can cover its customers to go to either hospital, so they ask each hospital what it would cost them. The insurer might not be so concerned about whether patients like the food or not; it has an incentive to think about issues more critical than meals. If both insurers and hospitals have to look at cost-containment when patients enter their systems, they have to analyze how much money they're spending, how much they may be wasting, and how low they can bid and still survive as a business. This would be a vastly different approach for hospital leadership to take. The insurer might even decide to cover both hospitals, with a lower co-pay when members go to the hospital that costs them less. Working together, hospital and physician leaders could creatively design a multitude of models to maintain a competitive environment and yet not over-regulate providers.

Rebalancing primary and specialty care

Healthcare reform must include the development of fair compensation that reflects real value and reduces payment discrepancies among physicians. While discrepancies have always existed within the physician community, the gulf has widened tremendously since the advent of higher reimbursements for doing procedures than for spending time with patients. When Medicare started reducing overall reimbursement with across-the-board cuts, it created incentives to do procedures rather than to see patients. Physicians who were trained to do well-reimbursed procedures became relatively wealthy, while physicians who were trained primarily to consult with patients fell way behind.

Consider the financial realities of cardiology versus primary care. Cardiologists are trained both to do procedures and to see patients. If they're proficient, cardiologists doing invasive procedures can do several of them in a short period of time and make a lot of money. A good cardiologist can make $15,000 a day in the catheterization lab, and other specialists can earn similar sums doing high-tech procedures. But a primary care doctor cannot possibly earn that kind of income by seeing patients in the office.

So specialists such as cardiologists become fairly wealthy and sub-specialists such as interventional cardiologists become even more so, while in areas such as Seattle – where Medicare and Medicaid reimbursement rates for patient visits are so low – primary care doctors are struggling just to pay back their medical school loans and survive in practice. Nurse practitioners in a private cardiology practice can earn more than primary care doctors in some communities.

Needless to say, such financial imbalances cause tremendous, often unspoken tensions within medicine, especially when the future of reimbursement is so uncertain. As a cardiologist I worked hard, but I wasn't forced to see 60 or 70 patients a day in the office to make ends meet, the way today's primary care doctors can be. And while invasive cardiologists talk about the stress of performing "life-and-death" procedures as part of the explanation for their high reimbursements, the reality is that most physicians enjoy the challenge of working in the catheterization lab. Although doing cardiac procedures can be stressful, I suspect it's not as stressful as dealing with 60 different patients in one day.

As physicians in different specialties, then, our daily lives have become vastly different. For an internist, it's hard to enjoy going to work when you have to see 60 patients that day, just plowing through, while patients are angry because you're not spending enough time with them or answering all of their questions. The irony is that the time pressures from low reimbursement in primary care can push patients toward seeing specialists more often. The specialist has more time, a beautiful office with a tropical aquarium and headsets for music, and a relaxed receptionist at the front desk with time to chat and calm patients' nerves. Specialists can afford to offer those luxuries, but it creates ill will among physicians and even inappropriate referring patterns between primary and specialty care. Some primary care doctors send patients to specialists because they don't have time to deal with them, while other primary care doctors try to prevent their patients from seeing specialists at all, out of fear that they'll never see those patients again.

We as a physician community need to come up with an algorithm to determine what our various professional services are worth and demand that all physicians are adequately reimbursed. But we also need to recognize that physicians can no longer earn a million dollars without producing a million dollars' worth of value. Although primary care doctors will likely continue to earn somewhat less than specialists since they spend fewer years in training with deferred income, the gap in reimbursement needs to close.

No doubt we now have too few primary care doctors in the system. To be successful in a future integrated system of care, physicians have to be comfortable with the other professionals they're working with and their place in the system. It's not fair for primary care doctors to feel like others are extremely well paid while they're working themselves to the bone and can't survive in practice. Needless to say, this rebalancing of primary and specialty care will be a huge challenge moving forward in the future. As we take a harder look at procedures and realize that the system is doing far more of them than are medically necessary and appropriate, there will be fewer procedures to do and possibly too many physicians trained to do them. Some of those specialists may have to start seeing more patients in the office and doing fewer procedures.

This issue has been debated in medical journals for years, where editorials and op-ed pieces agree that medicine has evolved into a fractured society. Internal medicine journals such as *The New England Journal of Medicine* and *Lancet* publish editorials about the need for more primary care doctors and better reimbursement for them. In contrast, specialty journals are filled with editorials about the need and benefits of doing even more procedures. It's hard to find common ground among the current factions of balkanized medicine, but that would be one of the critical tasks for future physician leaders.

Changing physician incentives

Hospitals today are forced to walk a fine line since they're so dependent on physicians for their revenue; most patients agree to go to whichever hospital their doctor sends them to. But hospitals must be circumspect about how they discuss referrals with physicians. Increasingly, the regulatory environment scrutinizes the relationship between physicians and hospitals, with tremendous sensitivity to the way hospitals communicate with doctors about referrals. It's against the law for hospitals to "buy" physician referrals due to federal regulations known as the "Stark Laws," which prohibit doctors from referring patients to entities in which they have financial interests.

On the other hand, hospital leaders need to be able to tell doctors what their organizations want and don't want them to do, to some degree, to keep their organizations viable. Hospitals now track what their various doctors are doing and give their physicians "score cards" showing their utilization of procedures and hospital resources compared to what their colleagues are doing, without revealing colleagues' names. The score cards typically compare factors such as the mean number of procedures doctors are doing and mean length-of-stay of their patients in the hospital.

How does this communication change physician behavior? It's subtle. Hospital executives don't want to see increases in length-of-stay because that's costly to the hospital, but on the other hand, the quantity of high-profit procedures is critical to their financial survival as an organization. As a physician, then, if I see that I did 100 cardiac catheterizations last month while my colleague did 350, what message would that give me? There's an upside to my income, should I choose to accept it. With the length-of-stay data, if I'm out of line with my colleagues, I'd realize that I'm not going to be the hospital's favorite doc for long. Again, financial incentives are at play, pulling at the hospital's bottom line. For procedures that generate money, hospital leaders want to see as many as possible performed; that's why they love cardiologists, orthopedic surgeons, and oncologists.

So while a hospital and its physician leaders may want to integrate care, there are huge regulatory and payment systems obstructing the way, including Medicare Parts A and B and how private insurers pay for these services. The government still pays hospitals a separate payment via Medicare Part A, while it pays the doctors a separate payment through Medicare Part B. Nearly everyone agrees that it's a fragmented, inefficient system. But how do we put an end to fragmented care with perverse incentives when we pay for it that way?

Successful healthcare reform – which would include the end of fee-for-service billing – will be bloody, but it has to happen. So let's allow the physicians to figure it out and incentivize them to do so. That's the only way to end the war among physicians about who earns what, to end the war between physicians and hospitals about who gets paid what, and to end the war among the other players in the system vying for their share of the pie. The goal is to create a healthcare culture where all factions see that they're sharing the pie and need to figure out how to do that together for the greater good.

Making the best use of clinical expertise

When hospital leaders make across-the-board cuts to improve the bottom line, they look at where they're spending the bulk of their money. Salaries for registered nurses (RNs) are one of the largest line items for hospitals; they're more expensive than LPNs, receptionists, and janitors, so hospitals typically ratchet down the number of RNs to cut costs. When nurses are unionized, hospitals can't pay them any less; they can only use fewer of them. Certainly, the patient's positive perception of the hospital drops with fewer qualified, tenured nurses to provide care, although the hospital "successfully" cut costs.

On the other hand, in a prospective system with bundled payments and a fixed amount of money, nurses as well as physicians would have input on how that budget would be divided, and the clinicians as a team could figure out ways to provide better care with fewer resources. As professionals, nurses could evaluate which tasks they really need to do themselves and which tasks they could delegate to a less-expensive caregiver. Rather than cutting more nurses from budgets, the goal would be to figure out how to use nurses and other caregivers more efficiently.

Especially during times of stress and change – which is the current climate in health care – people need to feel secure that they can participate in reform without eliminating their own jobs. That's a key factor in a new culture of health care: People need to feel that they are buying into an admirable mission as part of a team and will be treated with respect.

Toward that end, healthcare organizations can draw upon successful corporate cultures in other industries as models for inspiration. When the U.S. retail market plummeted recently, for instance, leadership at Nordstrom, a family-owned retailer, told all of its employees that they'd do their best not to let anyone go, but that people would have to work harder and perhaps even take a pay cut until business improved. Throughout those turbulent times, the staff worked hard and successfully avoided layoffs. That kind of culture builds an incredible amount of loyalty and satisfies many of the intangible psychological needs to belong, to be treated with respect, and to be part of something bigger than oneself. It may take awhile, but the healthcare industry can arrive there, too, with physician leaders as key players in that transition.

Designing clinical pathways with measurable value

A key role for physicians in cost-containment will be to develop disease-management pathways that provide measurable value. Because of the subtlety of evaluating the science behind evidence-based medicine, physicians – rather than bureaucrats – are in the best position to determine how to provide measurable value and recommend clinical pathways that work while eliminating those that don't.

Outcomes data from clinical trials typically falls into one of several categories, informed in part by whether the data comes from multiple, well-controlled, randomized clinical trials. In the current culture of the autonomous physician mindset, physicians use this information any way they choose, while in a more collaborative, integrated system, a team of physicians would use the data to agree on more consistent decision-making and clinical pathways for treatment.

With one category of outcomes data, there is clear evidence that a treatment, such as a drug, can be safe and effective and its benefits outweigh its risks, based on several well-controlled, randomized clinical trials. Perhaps surprisingly for consumers, a minority of treatments falls into this category. Physicians know that certain antibiotics, for instance, are the drug of choice for a hospital-acquired pneumonia and that other antibiotics are the drug of choice for a community-acquired pneumonia; the dose, duration of treatment, and monitoring has been well established. In cardiology, we know that beta blockers are the drug of choice after an acute myocardial infarction (heart attack), ACE inhibitors are the drug of choice for patients with congestive heart failure, and people who have had a coronary event such as a heart attack have better outcomes on statins. For this category of treatment, the evidence is clear, the data overwhelmingly positive.

But looking at the realities of how physicians apply that information clinically, perhaps only a quarter of all patients are benefiting from it right now. The issue is an inconsistent application of data. Even in the category of outcomes research where there's irrefutable proof that a given treatment works, physicians may or may not be prescribing according to the data, in part because of the physician culture of autonomy. It may run contrary to popular understanding, but the practice of medicine still relies heavily on individual prescribing patterns and habits of doctors, at times even more so than on accumulated scientific data. Here again is a clear arena for future physician leaders to have a tremendous impact on quality of care, and cost-effectiveness of care, in America.

With another category of outcomes research, there is irrefutable evidence that a treatment is harmful. Using calcium channel blockers in patients with coronary disease and heart failure is not a good idea, nor is putting people on aspirin instead of the anticoagulant Coumadin (warfarin) for atrial fibrillation. Using broad-spectrum antibiotics when a specific antibiotic or no antibiotic is indicated has negative long-term effects for both patients and for society. The issue for healthcare reform – and for physician leaders – is why society continues to reimburse for treatment that a doctor orders, when we know those treatments have harmful outcomes?

Nearly as problematic, from a systemic perspective, is the category of treatment that, while not proven harmful, has no proven benefit, such as inserting stents in patients in the absence of acute heart attack or uncontrolled symptoms. Without clear data on improved longevity and morbidity, why are we as physicians performing so many stent procedures, and why are we as a society paying for them? Think of the millions of dollars in savings if we were to reconsider the clinical protocols for that one procedure.

Whatever the science and clear data behind a given treatment, physicians tend to hold their ground on knowing what's best for their patients; and insurers don't want to go to war with doctors over that. Trying to regulate treatment, for insurers, has always been a losing proposition, whether they comb through every case of utilization after the fact with an expensive bureaucracy or try to regulate before the fact, asking doctors to fill out paperwork to preauthorize every treatment decision they make. Insurers might send the doctor a challenging letter or two and occasionally deny payment, but that's about it.

In the future, physicians working together in an integrated, prospective payment system could feel free to question each other about treatment choices, especially for those clinical pathways that weren't offering enough value to patients but were costing a lot of money. A doctor would have a tough time defending those practices to trained colleagues who see that wasting money decreases their ability to deliver a high quality of care because it squanders a limited resource and ultimately flows out of their own pockets. That would be a different game, a new decision-making environment. It highlights another benefit in bringing physician leadership into hospitals: to overcome resistance among staff physicians to using more consistent clinical pathways that lead to better patient outcomes and more streamlined, cost-effective care.

Integrated care: a new model of prospective payment

Too few healthcare analysts and policy makers are challenging the root of the fee-for-service mentality to change it – for example, toward a prospective payment system. I'd argue that we should prospectively pay for patient populations, and let the physicians, hospitals, nurses, pharmacists, and other providers in a geographic area figure out for themselves how to best utilize those dollars. In a prospective payment system, a single, fixed payment would be made for all medical services related to that consumer. With the right reforms, the prospective payment model could be used not only in hospitals but in future integrated healthcare systems, made up of hospitals plus multiple types of clinicians, specialists, and subspecialists, to take care of populations in a region on a per-patient, per-month basis. This degree of integration would require a new level of effective physician leadership.

A prospective payment system would be similar to managed care organizations that are self-insured, such as Kaiser Permanente in California and Group Health in Washington. But instead of Kaiser or Group Health competing with systems using a fee-for-service model, they would now compete on a more level playing field with all systems using a prepaid, per-patient, per-year financial model. In this new model, competition among prospectively paid providers would spurn the creation of value in health care. The providers who offer the most comprehensive care at the lowest cost would set the bar for others in the market. Rather than a prospective payment system with financial incentives to limit care, then, this integrated care model would involve a group of providers collaborating as one entity to cover all aspects of care. If we figure out how to deliver the highest value care, we can more rationally decide how to share the funding pie.

When payments to an integrated healthcare delivery system cover a patient's entire "care episode," it creates an incentive for providers to work together, avoid duplication, and prevent unnecessary utilization of care. More importantly, having integrated systems competing against other integrated systems levels the playing field in the healthcare market, eliminating huge discrepancies among winners and losers in health care. As it stands today, physicians can leave an organization such as Group Health and double or triple their salaries. A diagnostic imaging company such as Siemens Healthcare can sell a surplus of scanners to independent providers because their use is disproportionately reimbursed by insurers, including Medicare. The more scanners sold, the higher the profit, not only to the seller, Siemens, but to the buyers – the hospitals and physicians who make money off procedures and testing – as well. Hypothetically, if there were instead only a few integrated healthcare systems in one city, all competing for a lump-sum payment to take care of that city's population, then the more unnecessary scanners each system bought that didn't add value, the lower its income and competitive position in the marketplace. So instead of an endless number of customers, a company like Siemens would now have just a few.

An integrated system could be similar to what Canada does, but without being a government-run program. A handful of private insurers could serve a given population base, and consumers could pick among them for their healthcare system: "I'm going with Premera insurance and Northwest Hospital physicians," or "I choose Blue Cross with Swedish Hospital doctors." Each consumer would choose an affiliation with a healthcare system that combines an insurance company with an integrated system – physicians, nurses, pharmacists, care extenders such as home health aides, a hospital, outpatient surgical center, long-term care facility – all working together under the same incentives to deliver high-quality, value-driven services across the continuum of care.

Each of those local, integrated systems would receive set revenue per year for each person who signs up to be taken care of in that system, and it would be up to that integrated system to figure out among all of their providers how to make it work financially. Part of the providers' incentive would be knowledge that at the end of the year, if their patients weren't satisfied, they'd change providers the next year. This prevents the control of a government-run system that could become a monopoly; consumers could always decide to go elsewhere for medical care, so local healthcare systems would have the pressures of competition with a level playing field of incentives.

The benefits of integrated systems

In an integrated delivery system, a group of providers collaborate to determine all of a patient's care and utilization of healthcare services, embracing the "continuum of care" – from the intensive care of the hospital through office visits to care in the home. No economic incentives exist to compete with other providers within the system; everyone is on the same team. One check can be written to cover everything that an integrated system provides to a patient in one episode of care. The realistic, long-term vision of integration accepts the idea of capitation and a single check, and accepts that fee-for-service is a dinosaur that won't work in a system trying to control overall costs for a national population. New, integrated systems could be self-insured, but integration wouldn't likely affect Medicare; politicians won't turn their backs on Medicare. Instead, integrated systems might have their own insurance product and contract with Medicare at competitive rates.

More consistent technology utilization is another benefit of integration, especially since the cost of most new technology is increasing, such as with titanium implants for joint replacement surgeries. Most decisions about what physicians currently use are autonomous, uncontrolled by the hospital. But if a steel hip works perfectly well in the vast majority of cases, why would an orthopedic surgeon order a titanium or platinum hip for all of their patients? In a cost-contained system, hospital leadership wouldn't order the more expensive implant unless medically indicated; the system wouldn't be able to support it. While each physician may have a favorite stent, pacemaker, or knee prosthesis, if physicians and hospitals work together in an integrated system with cost-containment in mind, then deciding which devices and drugs to stock in the hospital would become significantly simpler, easier, and more cost-effective.

Determining clinically useful data

As a society, we're in an information explosion – and perhaps in no other arena as much as in health care. We're so wed to having limitless information that we don't realize that too much information itself can be paralyzing and distracting, especially when that data has no useful purpose. The upside is great with the Genome Project, for instance; but after genetic testing is done, then what? For a while physicians offered full-body CT scans, and what they found were multiple, incidental, anatomical "abnormalities," which turned out to have no clinical significance whatsoever – yet were leading doctors and patients to intervene when the intervention was much worse than doing nothing. As physicians, we're constantly looking for data, but there's also a point where we all need to use common sense about what we're doing. We need to step back and ask, "What are the realistic possibilities down this road for this data, and is it clinically useful?"

What can no longer be ignored in the healthcare reform conversation is the issue of physician utilization of resources. Consumers may worry about how much money doctors make; but in the healthcare economy of today, how much money doctors earn is hardly relevant. The real issue is how much money they have control over – their utilization of healthcare resources.

The most dangerous instrument in the medical armamentarium is the doctor's pen. As physicians, we can order expensive tests, expensive drugs, and expensive surgeries and hospitalizations. A single cardiologist can drive $40 to $50 million or more of utilization per year. Not enough physicians, consumers, and policy makers are paying attention to the reality of utilization as a major factor in healthcare reform. Developing effective physician leaders and employing more of them throughout the system would help resolve issues of clinically useful data and clinical value in procedures to avoid the costly waste in unnecessary overutilization. Physician leadership in creating value in health care is the only remaining, viable alternative to a government-run, single-party-payer system driven by bureaucracy.

Selected Bibliography

American Medical Association. The Medicare Physician Payment Schedule.
http://www.ama-assn.org/ama/pub/physician-resources/solutions-managing-your-practice/coding-billing-insurance/medicare/the-medicare-physician-payment-schedule.page?

American Medical Association. "Student Debt Statistics."
http://www.ama-assn.org/ama/pub/about-ama/our-people/member-groups-sections/medical-student-section/advocacy-policy/medical-student-debt/background.page?

Anstett, Patricia. "Canadians visit U.S. to get health care." Detroit Free Press, August 20, 2009.
http://www.freep.com/article/20090820/BUSINESS06/908200420/Canadians-visit-U-S-get-health-care

Appleby, Julie. "Costs of Employer Insurance Plans Surge in 2011." Kaiser Health News, September 27, 2011.
http://www.kaiserhealthnews.org/Stories/2011/September/27/Employer-Health-Coverage-Survey-Shows-Employer-Spending-Spike.aspx

Atlas, Scott. "10 Surprising Facts about American Health Care." National Center for Policy Analysis, March 24, 2009.
http://fraser.stlouisfed.org/publications/erp/page/8649/download/47455/8649_ERP.pdf

Beck, AH. "The Flexner Report and the Standardization of American Medicine." The Journal of the American Medical Association, 2004; 291(17):2139-2140.
http://jama.ama-assn.org/content/291/17/2139.full

Bodenheimer MD, Thomas. "Primary Care – Will It Survive?" New England Journal of Medicine, 2006; 355:861-864
http://www.nejm.org/doi/full/10.1056/NEJMp068155

Bradford, Harry. "America's 10 Best-Paying Professions: Bureau of Labor Statistics." The Huffington Post, May 21, 2011.
http://www.huffingtonpost.com/2011/05/20/top-ten-highest-paid-jobs_n_864907.html#s281484&title=10_Psychiatrists

Brown, BG et al. American Journal of Cardiology. 2001 July 19;88(2A):23E-26E.
http://www.ncbi.nlm.nih.gov/pubmed/11473741

Bybee, Roger. "The Doctors' Revolt." The American Prospect. July 1, 2008.
http://prospect.org/article/doctors-revolt

Center on Budget and Policy Priorities. "Policy Basics: Where Do Our Federal Tax Dollars Go?"
http://www.cbpp.org/cms/index.cfm?fa=view&id=1258

Center for Medicare & Medicaid Innovation. "Bundled Payments for Care Improvement."
http://innovations.cms.gov/initiatives/bundled-payments/index.html

Centers for Medicare & Medicaid Services. "National Health Expenditure Data."

https://www.cms.gov/NationalHealthExpendData/25_NHE_Fact_Sheet.asp

Centers for Medicare & Medicaid Services. "Shared Savings Program."
http://www.cms.gov/sharedsavingsprogram/

Centers for Medicare & Medicaid Services, Office of the Actuary. "National Health Expenditure Projections 2008-2018."
http://www.cms.gov/Research-Statistics-Data-and-Systems/Statistics-Trends-and-Reports/NationalHealthExpendData/downloads/proj2008.pdf

Congressional Budget Office. "The Long-Term Budget Outlook." June 25, 2009.
http://www.cbo.gov/ftpdocs/102xx/doc10297/chapter2.5.1.shtml

Congressional Budget Office. "Testimony on Fraud, Waste, and Abuse in Medicare." July 31, 1995.
http://www.cbo.gov/doc.cfm?index=5497&type=0

Connelly, Julie. "Doctors Are Opting Out of Medicare." *The New York Times,* **April 1, 2009.**
http://www.nytimes.com/2009/04/02/business/retirementspecial/02health.html

Crutsinger, Martin. "Obama Sends FY2013 Budget Proposals to Congress." The Associated Press/*Businessweek***, February 13, 2012.**
http://www.businessweek.com/ap/financialnews/D9SSJSNO0.htm

Demaerschalk MD, Bart M and Durocher, Donna L. "How Diagnosis-Related Group 559 Will Change the U.S. Medicare

Cost Reimbursement Ratio for Stroke Centers," Stroke: Journal of the American Heart Association. 2007;38: 1309-1312.
http://stroke.ahajournals.org/content/38/4/1309.full.pdf

Dorn, Stan and Buettgens, Matthew. "Net Effects of the Affordable Care Act on State Budgets." The Urban Institute, December 2010.
http://www.urban.org/UploadedPDF/1001480-Affordable-Care-Act.pdf

Emanuel, Ezekiel J. "Saving by the Bundle." The New York Times. November 16, 2011.
http://opinionator.blogs.nytimes.com/2011/11/16/saving-by-the-bundle/

Emanuel, Ezekiel J. "Spending More Doesn't Make Us Healthier." The New York Times. October 27, 2011.
http://opinionator.blogs.nytimes.com/2011/10/27/spending-more-doesnt-make-us-healthier/

Feeny, David et al. "Comparing Population Health in the United States and Canada." Population Health Metrics, 2010, 8:8 (29 April 2010).
http://www.pophealthmetrics.com/content/8/April/2010

Fonarow, GC et al. "Impact of a Comprehensive Heart Failure Management Program on Hospital Readmission and Functional Status of Patients with Advanced Heart Failure." Journal of the American College of Cardiology, 1997;30:725-732.
http://content.onlinejacc.org/cgi/content/short/30/3/725

George Washington University: National Health Policy Forum. "The Basics: Relative Value Units (RVUs)." February 12, 2009.
http://www.nhpf.org/library/the-basics/Basics_RVUs_02-12-09.pdf

Goodnough, Abby and Sack, Kevin. "Massachusetts Tries to Rein in Its Health Costs." October 17, 2011.
http://www.nytimes.com/2011/10/18/us/massachusetts-tries-to-rein-in-its-health-care-cost.html?_r=1&hp

Gould, Elise. "2010 Marks Another Year of Decline for Employer-Sponsored Health Insurance Coverage." Economic Policy Institute, September 13, 2011.
http://www.epi.org/publication/2010-marks-year-decline-employer-sponsored/

Gruber, PhD, Jonathan. "The Role of Consumer Copayments for Health Care: Lessons from the RAND Health Insurance Experiment and Beyond." Kaiser Family Foundation, October 2006.
http://www.kff.org/insurance/upload/7566.pdf

Harding, Anne. "Heart Stents Used Twice as Often in U.S. vs. Canada." Reuters, June 15, 2010.
http://www.reuters.com/article/2010/06/15/us-heart-stents-id USTRE65E60220100615

Harris, Gardiner. "Doctor Faces Suits Over Cardiac Stents." The New York Times, December 5, 2010.
http://www.nytimes.com/2010/12/06/health/06stent.html?scp=1&sq=midei&st=cse

Health Council of Canada. "Decisions, Decisions: Family Doctors as Gatekeepers to Prescription Drugs and Diagnostic Imaging in Canada." September 2010.
http://www.scribd.com/doc/38226497/Decisions-decisions

Hoover, Donald R et al. "Medical Expenditures in the Last Year of Life." Health Services Research, 2002 December; 37(6):1625-1642.
http://www.ncbi.nlm.nih.gov/pmc/articles/PMC1464043/

Iglehart, John K. "Medicare Payment Reform – Proposals for Paying for an SGR Repeal." The New England Journal of Medicine, 2011;365:1859-1861.
http://www.nejm.org/doi/full/10.1056/NEJMp1111954

Jha MD, Ashish K et al. "Use of Electronic Health Records in U.S. Hospitals." New England Journal of Medicine, 2009; 360:1628-1638.
http://www.nejm.org/doi/full/10.1056/NEJMsa0900592

Johnson, T. "Healthcare Costs and U.S. Competitiveness." Council on Foreign Relations, March 26, 2012.
http://www.cfr.org/health-science-and-technology/healthcare-costs-us-competitiveness/p13325

Kaiser Family Foundation. "Employer Health Benefits 2011 Annual Survey." September 27, 2011.
http://ehbs.kff.org/

Kaiser Family Foundation. "Focus on Health Reform: Summary of New Health Reform Law." April 15, 2011.
http://www.kff.org/healthreform/upload/8061.pdf

Kaiser Family Foundation: Health Reform Source. "CMS Actuaries Release New Health Spending Projections." September 9, 2010.
http://healthreform.kff.org/scan/2010/september/cms-actuaries-release-new-health-spending-projections.aspx

Kaiser Family Foundation. "Medicare Now and in the Future." October 2, 2008.
http://www.kff.org/medicare/h08_7821.cfm

Kaiser Family Foundation. "The Most Popular Provision in the ACA." Kaiser Family Foundation Health Tracking Poll, conducted November 2011.
http://www.kff.org/pullingittogether/Most-Popular-Provision-ACA.cfm

Kaiser Family Foundation. "Side-by-Side Comparison of Major Health Care Reform Proposals."
http://www.kff.org/healthreform/sidebyside.cfm

Kaushal MD, MPH, Rainu et al. "Return on Investment for a Computerized Physician Order Entry System." Journal of the American Medical Informatics Association, 2006 May-June; 13(3):261-266.
http://www.sciencedirect.com/science/article/pii/S106750270600020X

Kavilanz, Parija. "U.S. will pay half of all health care costs by 2020." CNN Money, July 28, 2011.
http://money.cnn.com/2011/07/28/news/economy/healthcare_spending_forecast/index.htm

Kocher, MD, Robert and Sahni, BS, Nikhil R. "Hospitals' Race to Employ Physicians – The Logic behind a Money-Losing Proposition." New England Journal of Medicine, 2011;364:1790-1793.
http://www.nejm.org/doi/full/10.1056/NEJMp1101959

Kravitz, RL and Bell, RA. "Direct-to-Consumer Advertising of Prescription Drugs: Balancing Benefits and Risks, and a Way

Forward." Clinical Pharmacology & Therapeutics, 82, 360-362 (October 2007).
http://www.nature.com/clpt/journal/v82/n4/full/6100348a.html

Levey, Noam N. "Democrats Drive Drop in Support for Healthcare Law in New Poll." Los Angeles Times, October 28, 2011.
http://articles.latimes.com/2011/oct/28/news/la-pn-health-poll-20111027

Liebowitz, Stan. "Policy Analysis: Why Health Care Costs Too Much." CATO Institute, June 23, 1994.
http://www.cato.org/pubs/pas/pa211.html

Massachusetts Medical Society. Making Sense of the Stark Law. 2005.
http://www.massmed.org/AM/Template.cfm?Section=Search§ion=PPRC_Regulatory_Compliance&template=/CM/ContentDisplay.cfm&ContentFileID=773

Morris, Lewis. Testimony for the U.S. Department of Health & Human Services on "Reducing Fraud, Waste, and Abuse in Medicare," before the U.S. House of Representatives on June 15, 2010.
http://www.hhs.gov/asl/testify/2010/06/t20100615c.html

National Priorities Project. "Year End Wrap-Up: One (Bumpy) Year in the Life of the Federal Budget." September 28, 2011.
http://nationalpriorities.org/en/publications/2011/year-end-wrap-up/?gclid=CPvGIKaiqqwCFQRShwod9iYH

NationMaster.com. "Health Statistics: Life Expectancy at Birth: Total Population (2011) by Country." Data from CIA World Factbooks, December 2003 to March 2011.

http://www.nationmaster.com/graph/hea_lif_exp_at_bir_tot_pop-life-expectancy-birth-total-population&date=2011

Office of the Inspector General, Region IX. Medicare Hospital Prospective Payment System: How DRG Rates Are Calculated and Updated. August 2001.
http://oig.hhs.gov/oei/reports/oei-09-00-00200.pdf

Office of the Legislative Counsel, 111th Congress. Compilation of Patient Protection and Affordable Care Act. May 2010.
http://docs.house.gov/energycommerce/ppacacon.pdf

Peterson, Chris L and Burton, Rachel. "Congressional Research Service Report for Congress: U.S. Health Care Spending: Comparison with Other OECD Countries." September 17, 2007.
http://assets.opencrs.com/rpts/RL34175_20070917.pdf

Radelat, Ana. "The Growing Ruckus Over the RUC and Medicare Fees." University of Pennsylvania, Leonard Davis Institute of Health Economics, LDI Health Economist, June 23, 2011.
http://ldihealtheconomist.com/he000009.shtml

Rampell, Catherine. "How Much Do Doctors in Other Countries Make?" The New York Times, May 31, 2012.
http://economix.blogs.nytimes.com/2009/07/15/how-much-do-doctors-in-other-countries-make/

Reznick, Ran. "Doctors Demand 60 Percent Raise." Haaretz Daily Newspaper, May 27, 2007.
http://www.haaretz.com/print-edition/business/doctors-demand-60-percent-raise-1.221487

Robert Wood Johnson Foundation. "Disease Management Program Reduces Hospital Days for Chronic Renal Disease Patients." May 2002.
http://www.rwjf.org/reports/grr/032061.htm

Rovner, Julie. "Medicare Can't Rescue Congress on Fix for Doctors' Pay." NPR: Shots, December 22, 2011.
http://www.npr.org/blogs/health/2011/12/22/144145493/medicare-cant-rescue-congress-on-fix-for-doctors-pay

Sahadi, Jeanne. "The Ugly Math of Medicare." CNN Money. April 8, 2011.
http://money.cnn.com/2011/04/07/news/economy/medicare_reform/index.htm?iid=EAL

Sibert, Karen S. "Don't Quit This Day Job." The New York Times, June 11, 2011.
http://www.nytimes.com/2011/06/12/opinion/12sibert.html?pagewanted=all

Starr, Paul. Remedy and Reaction: The Peculiar American Struggle over Health Care Reform. New Haven: Yale University Press, 2011.

Starr, Paul. The Logic of Healthcare Reform. Whittle Communications, Grand Rounds Press. 1992.

Starr, Paul. The Social Transformation of American Medicine: The Rise of a Sovereign Profession and the Making of a Vast Industry. New York: Basic Books, 1982.

Stockdale, Holly. Congressional Research Service: "Medicare Program Integrity: Activities to Protect Medicare from Payment Errors, Fraud, and Abuse." March 15, 2010.

http://aging.senate.gov/crs/medicare18.pdf

Tulshyan, Ruchika. "Primary-Care Doctors: Saying No to $191,000 a Year." Time Magazine, August 22, 2010.
http://www.time.com/time/business/article/0,8599,2012443,00.html

U.S. Census Bureau. The Next Four Decades: The Older Population in the United States: 2010 to 2050. May 2010.
http://www.census.gov/prod/2010pubs/p25-1138.pdf

U.S. Department of Labor: Bureau of Labor Statistics. "Economic News Release: Employer Costs for Employee Compensation," March 14, 2012.
http://www.bls.gov/news.release/ecec.nr0.htm

U.S. Department of Labor: Bureau of Labor Statistics. "Occupational Outlook Handbook: Physicians and Surgeons."
http://www.bls.gov/ooh/Healthcare/Physicians-and-surgeons.htm

Van de Water, Paul N. "The Sustainable Growth Rate Formula and Health Reform." Center on Budget and Policy Priorities, April 21, 2010.
http://www.cbpp.org/cms/index.cfm?fa=view&id=3166

Ventola, CL. "Challenges in Evaluating and Standardizing Medical Devices in Health Care Facilities." Pharmacy and Therapeutics, June 2008;v.33(6):348-359.
http://www.ncbi.nlm.nih.gov/pmc/articles/PMC2683611/

Worstall, Tim. "What Bomb Buried in Obamacare?" Forbes, December 3, 2011.
http://www.forbes.com/sites/timworstall/2011/12/03/what-bomb-buried-in-obamacare/

Wright, Caroline. "The Rise and Rise of Stents." Scrip Magazine: Pharmaceutical Issues in Perspective, January 2006. http://www.cambridgeconsultants.com/downloads/articles/Scrip_06_01_LRes.pdf

www.ingramcontent.com/pod-product-compliance
Lightning Source LLC
Chambersburg PA
CBHW051453170526
45166CB00001B/228

9781477640470